BEGINNING REFLECTIVE PRACTICE
SECOND EDITION

Melanie Jasper

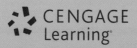

CENGAGE
Learning

Australia • Brazil • Canada • Mexico • Singapore • Spain • United Kingdom • United States

**CENGAGE
Learning**

**Beginning Reflective Practice,
Second Edition**
Melanie Jasper

Publishing Director: Linden Harris

Commissioning Editor: Annabel Ainscow

Production Editor: Beverley Copland

Production Controller: Eyvett Davis

Marketing Manager: Lauren Mottram

Typesetter: Integra Software
Services Pvt. Ltd.

Cover design: Adam Renvoize

For product information and technology assistance,
contact **emea.info@cengage.com.**

For permission to use material from this text or product,
and for permission queries,
email **emea.permissions@cengage.com.**

British Library Cataloguing-in-Publication Data
A catalogue record for this book is available from the British Library.

ISBN: 978-1-4080-7487-9

Cengage Learning EMEA
Cheriton House, North Way, Andover, Hampshire, SP10 5BE,
United Kingdom

Cengage Learning products are represented in Canada by Nelson Education Ltd.

For your lifelong learning solutions, visit **www.cengage.co.uk**

Purchase your next print book, e-book or e-chapter at
www.cengagebrain.com

Printed in Singapore by Seng Lee Press
1 2 3 4 5 6 7 8 9 10 – 15 14 13

CONTENTS

ACKNOWLEDGEMENTS

I would like to thank the students, lecturers and practitioners who made the first edition of this book such a success, and the need for a second edition. I hope this book confirms reflective practice as a 'way of being' for a health care practitioner; that it testifies to the development of practitioners as truly embedded in reflexively interacting with their environment, to provide the best possible health care for their patients and clients.

The publishers would like to thank Alison Clarke, Dr Sue Higham, Dr Jennifer Loke, Dr Jenny Moore and Fawzia Zaida for their insightful review comments on the manuscript and Dr Clare Hopkinson for mapping the chapters to the NMC (2010) standards and essential skills clusters.

ABOUT THE AUTHOR

Melanie Jasper is Professor of Nursing and Head of the College of Human and Health Sciences, Swansea University. Previously a Health Visitor and Midwife, Melanie entered nurse education at the time of its transition into Higher Education. She has been involved in educational, curricula and practice development for more than 20 years, helping practitioners develop critical thinking and reflective skills for practice at all academic levels, as well as working in practice environments to encourage work-based learning approaches. She has written six books in the areas of reflective practice and professional development, and has published numerous academic papers and chapters in books on the same topic over the past 20 years. She has been editor of the *Journal of Nursing Management* (Wiley) for ten years, and led its development to achieving first ranking in the impact factor assessment in 2010 and coming 13/88 in the nursing science category. In 2011, Melanie was appointed Adjunct Professor to the University of Ilorin in Nigeria to help developed under-graduate and graduate nursing and social work programmes. In 2012 she worked with the Welsh Government on the Professionalism in Nursing and Midwifery project, which aims to raise the visibility of high quality nursing care and provide supportive and developmental mechanisms for all practitioners at work. Melanie's work is noted for being accessible in style, and in enabling readers to understand and apply theoretical principles to practice. Hence, she was asked to write the first edition of this text.

Series Editors for the *Nursing and Health Care Practice* Series:

Dr Lynne Wigens, Director of Nursing and Quality at The Ipswich Hospital NHS Trust. Visiting Senior Fellow University Campus Suffolk

Dr Jane Day, Head of Division, Practice Learning and Midwifery, School of Nursing and Midwifery, University Campus Suffolk

INTRODUCTION

In this book I introduce you to the concept of reflective practice – what it is and why it is important, both as a strategy for your own learning and for developing your professional practice. You can then approach the rest of the book with an understanding of what you are trying to achieve in developing strategies for your own learning from practice experiences. I also use this section to introduce the rest of the book to you.

Nobody comes to learning as a blank slate; we all have a wealth of knowledge and experiences that form a springboard for developing new and exciting roles and skills. As a fledgling professional, you will be faced with what might, at the moment, seem like a daunting array and amount of learning. This comes firstly from both the hard slog of learning facts and accepted knowledge, and secondly from acquiring and practising the physical skills of your profession with confidence, so that they become second nature. As you start to tick these off your list, you will find that other elements of professional practice start to creep into your consciousness. You will meet professional codes of conduct, and ethics. These underpin the ways in which you form relationships with your clients and enable us to do things to them that under other circumstances would be seen as beyond normal interaction with strangers – things such as touching, asking personal questions, or expecting people to reveal parts of their bodies to us that would normally remain covered. Many of these areas will be considered by looking at how you communicate with others and explaining how to form professional relationships that are 'common knowledge' because of the unspoken boundaries accepted by both the professional and the client.

We can often only learn these things by observing others, being placed in the situation ourselves and building up experiences that we can draw on.

And this is where reflective practice comes in. The ideas and strategies that you meet in this book are designed to help you become aware of this professional development in the third area of knowledge and skills. You will need these skills when you finally graduate from your course and are entitled to be called a professional. Reflective skills, particularly structured reflective strategies, enable us to make the most of everything that we do. This includes not only remembering things that have already happened but also anticipating and planning for the future.

In Chapter 1, 'What is reflective practice?', I set the scene of reflective practice, exploring what it is and why you will need it as a strategy for learning from your professional experience. I introduce you to the basic theories underpinning reflective practice and explore the key concepts within it in detail. This chapter provides you with the foundation for understanding what reflective practice is and why it is important.

In Chapter 2, 'Knowing ourselves', I start you off using reflective techniques. The first section in this chapter will help you identify your own strengths and weaknesses and start you thinking about how you can make the most of these as you proceed through your course. In the second section I ask you to think about the professional values that will underpin your practice, and where these come from. The next section looks at your learning style, with the last section identifying your approaches to writing. These last two sections will help you think about the ways in which you learn most effectively, and how you can plan to use these through your course and in your continuing development as a practitioner.

Chapter 3, 'Frameworks for reflection', presents three frameworks for reflective practice that can be used to structure your reflective activities. These are fully illustrated to help you see concrete examples of the ways in which they have helped other students to learn. These are fundamental in reflective practice as they provide a starting point for understanding what reflective cycles and processes involve. They provide a useful initial structure for reflective activities that you may then decide to build upon in the future.

In Chapter 4, 'Entering the working environment', I explore your role within the clinical environment and how you can use reflective practice to learn in it. Working environments offer you unique experiences that, unlike classroom learning, need to be explored and reinforced if you are to learn from them. It is easy to go through a day in practice without acknowledging the learning experiences that occur or ensuring that you identify your achievements. This chapter looks at maximizing your learning opportunities and making the most of what is available in different environments.

Chapter 5, 'Ways of reflecting on your own' and Chapter 6, 'Ways of reflecting with others', consider the different ways in which you can reflect by yourself or with other people. I look in depth at the advantages and challenges to both approaches, and raise issues to help you to explore the ways in which you can create opportunities and strategies for reflection. Chapter 5 focuses on strategies that you can use by yourself and includes sections on working with your learning style and thinking through your experiences. Most of the reflection you do will be by yourself and will not occur in a formal way at all. I try to get you thinking about how you can acknowledge this reflective work, whether it occurs while you are in practice or after the event. The majority of this chapter is devoted to exploring strategies for reflective writing in some depth. The purpose of this is to help you to think about your own attitudes about writing and to plan to use writing as a way of learning for yourself.

Chapter 6 focuses on the strategies that you can use when reflecting with others, especially those whose role it is to help you in your learning, such as your supervisors and lecturers. Reflecting with others has a different character from reflecting by yourself because you are essentially making your own unique experiences public. Reflecting with others is very powerful as a strategy for learning because you are able to draw on the perspectives that others bring to a situation. But this brings with it roles and responsibilities for all concerned to ensure that reflection is carried out in safety. This chapter identifies the issues that need to be considered before starting a reflective relationship with another person, so that maximum benefit can be gained by all those involved.

USING THIS BOOK TO DEVELOP SKILLS FOR REFLECTIVE PRACTICE

Throughout the book I will be providing you with tips and pointers so that the decisions you make about your own reflective practice can be informed ones that you make consciously. I present the issues that you need to consider about each of the topics covered, in the hope that this will enable you to use reflective techniques effectively as a strategy for your own learning.

This book aims to be both an introduction to reflective practice and a practical guide to help you to develop strategies and skills to begin your career as a reflective practitioner. Reflective practice is a technique for learning from experience that is applicable to all students in health care professions. I have used a range of examples throughout the book to illustrate the ideas being presented to you. Some of these arise from specific disciplines, such as nursing or physiotherapy, while others are the sorts of thing that could happen to anyone. The purpose of using examples from practice is to show you how a raw experience can be used as data for analysis and reflection to help you to learn and take action. The focus of the example itself is therefore not really relevant. So, if you are a student operating department practitioner, for instance, use the examples for the general point they are trying to convey rather than for the discipline they are drawn from.

Reflective practice is a deliberate activity – you have to take a decision to focus *deliberately* on something specific in order to learn from it. Throughout this book you will find a range of activities designed to help you develop the skills and strategies for reflective practice, by actually doing it. To get the most out of this book, it is worth taking the time to pick up pen and paper, create a file on your computer, or find other people to reflect with, while you work through the activities. Although reading the book will help you explore and understand what reflective practice is, the bottom line is that you can only learn from doing it yourself – there will be no miraculous transmission of skills, strategies and ideas from this book to your head! So, even if you are tempted to skip over the activities, do read them through and think about what they are asking you to do. At least come up with skeleton answers, even if you do not want to commit them to paper/computer file in the first instance.

In this book I take the approach that learning is not a passive exercise. I assume that the most effective and enjoyable way to learn from written material is to interact with what you are reading. So, I offer you several different ways of doing this, as I ask you to play with the ideas and consider what you are reading in the light of your own experiences.

I hope that you will enjoy learning to be a reflective practitioner with the help of the ideas and techniques presented through this book. It aims to be a practical guide and introduction to reflective practice for those starting out on the road of becoming health care practitioners. I wish you success in your learning and in your future career in working with other people to improve their lives and their experience of the health care system. The book is also in line with the current vision and strategy of Jane Cummings, Chief Nursing Officer for England, that Nurses, Midwives and Care-Givers should have the following 'Six Cs' values to unite their professions: care; compassion; competence; communication; courage and commitment.

WALK THROUGH TOUR

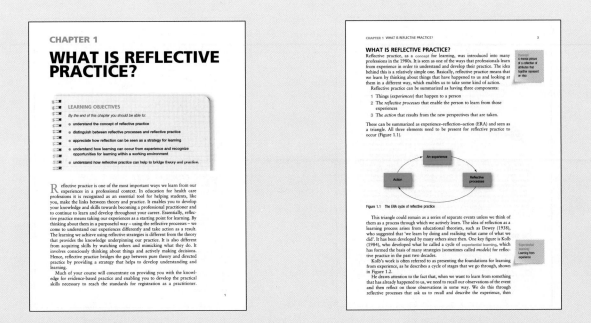

Learning outcomes: Listed at the beginning of each chapter, these emphasize the key topics that need to be understood before progressing to the next chapter.

Key word definitions: These are succinct definitions in the margin for important terms that are highlighted in the text.

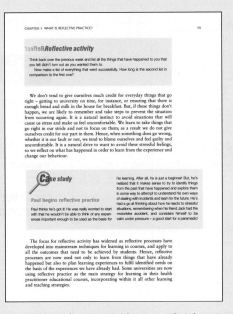

Reflective activity: An opportunity to undertake structured reflection on the topics under discussion.

Over to you: This feature encourages you to to think about how what you have just read relates to you and your experiences. You may be asked to think about what you will actually do with what you have just learned or discovered.

Case study: These are drawn from students' real-life experiences to demonstrate scenarios and encourage you to think about how you practice and learn.

Key points: You will find these at the end of sections to remind you of the main points made or provide a summary of the ideas that have been presented.

Rapid recap: At the end of each chapter, these give you the opportunity to test your understanding of the key issues raised. Answers are provided in the appendix.

DIGITAL RESOURCES

Dedicated Instructor Resources

To discover the dedicated instructor online
support resources accompanying this textbook,
instructors should register here for access:
http://login.cengage.com
Resources include:

- Teaching Tips
- PowerPoint slides

Online Student Resources

Instructor access

Instructors can access the online student resources by registering at
http://login.cengage.com or by speaking to their local
Cengage Learning EMEA representative.

Instructor resources

Instructors can use the integrated Engagement Tracker to track students' preparation and
engagement. The tracking tool can be used to monitor progress of the class as a whole, or for
individual students.

Student access

Students can access the online platform using the unique personal access card included in the
front of the book.

Student resources

A range of interactive learning tools tailored to *Beginning Reflective Practice* are available on the
online platform, including:

- Interactive eBook
- Case studies and questions
- Games and quizzes
- Glossary

- Critical Thinking Questions and Discussion
  Questions
- Flashcards and more

CHAPTER 1

WHAT IS REFLECTIVE PRACTICE?

LEARNING OBJECTIVES

By the end of this chapter you should be able to:

● understand the concept of reflective practice

● distinguish between reflective processes and reflective practice

● appreciate how reflection can be seen as a strategy for learning

● understand how learning can occur from experience and recognize opportunities for learning within a working environment

● understand how reflective practice can help to bridge theory and practice.

Reflective practice is one of the most important ways we learn from our experiences in a professional context. In education for health care professions it is recognized as an essential tool for helping students, like you, make the links between theory and practice. It enables you to develop your knowledge and skills towards becoming a professional practitioner and to continue to learn and develop throughout your career. Essentially, reflective practice means taking our experiences as a starting point for learning. By thinking about them in a purposeful way – using the reflective processes – we come to understand our experiences differently and take action as a result. The learning we achieve using reflective strategies is different from the theory that provides the knowledge underpinning our practice. It is also different from acquiring skills by watching others and mimicking what they do. It involves consciously thinking about things and actively making decisions. Hence, reflective practice bridges the gap between pure theory and directed practice by providing a strategy that helps to develop understanding and learning.

Much of your course will concentrate on providing you with the knowledge for evidence-based practice and enabling you to develop the practical skills necessary to reach the standards for registration as a practitioner.

However, there is a third element that you need to work on. It integrates theory and practice and helps you to become a responsible professional, aware of your own knowledge and skills, as well as your limitations, so that you are both competent and safe in your practice. This third area is complex, because it involves developing the critical analytical skills, thinking and judgement that allow you to make decisions. It can only arise from encountering different situations in the real world of practice. One of the most important ways you will do this is through reflective practice. The skills of reflective practice, together with the practical skills and underpinning knowledge base of your profession, learned during the foundations of your professional education, will stay with you, becoming part of who you are as a practitioner. Reflective learning is probably the most significant way that you will develop your practice once you have qualified.

Paul

Paul is an 18-year-old paramedic student who has just started his course. He sees a series of sessions on his timetable entitled 'Becoming a Reflective Practitioner', as part of his module on 'Being a Professional Practitioner' and is curious as to what this means. He thought he was in University to learn theory and do some practical work in the simulation laboratory. He was looking forward to his first placement with the Ambulance crew once he'd passed his first practical assessments. But, he'd never heard of reflective practice at all and couldn't really anticipate what it was about. It all sounded a bit nebulous, and, to some extent, challenging. Paul was quite prepared to be a passive learner – tell him what he needed to know, show him what he needed to do and he'd be okay. But, 'reflective' practitioner? At this early stage? Paul thought perhaps he'd better find out a bit more and did a Google search that night. He was astonished to find that learning to be a professional takes a great deal more personal activity and energy than he had thought, and that much of this related to him taking responsibility for his own learning through the experiences he would encounter during his education.

Over to you

How much have you thought, at this stage in your student career, about how you will learn to apply theory to practice, and to deal with situations that you have not previously encountered? Conversely, how do you think the learning you gain in practice placements will help you make sense of the theories you will need to learn?

Jot down a few ways that you might overcome these challenges in order to relate theory to practice and practice to theory.

WHAT IS REFLECTIVE PRACTICE?

Reflective practice, as a concept for learning, was introduced into many professions in the 1980s. It is seen as one of the ways that professionals learn from experience in order to understand and develop their practice. The idea behind this is a relatively simple one. Basically, reflective practice means that we learn by thinking about things that have happened to us and looking at them in a different way, which enables us to take some kind of action.

> **Concept**
> A mental picture of a collection of attributes that together represent an idea

Reflective practice can be summarized as having three components:

1 Things (*experiences*) that happen to a person
2 The *reflective processes* that enable the person to learn from those experiences
3 The *action* that results from the new perspectives that are taken.

These can be summarized as experience–reflection–action (ERA) and seen as a triangle. All three elements need to be present for reflective practice to occur (Figure 1.1).

Figure 1.1   The ERA cycle of reflective practice

This triangle could remain as a series of separate events unless we think of them as a process through which we actively learn. The idea of reflection as a learning process arises from educational theorists, such as Dewey (1938), who suggested that 'we learn by doing and realising what came of what we did'. It has been developed by many others since then. One key figure is Kolb (1984), who developed what he called a cycle of experiential learning, which has formed the basis of many strategies (sometimes called *models*) for reflective practice in the past two decades.

> **Experiential learning**
> Learning from experience

Kolb's work is often referred to as presenting the foundations for learning from experience, as he describes a cycle of stages that we go through, shown in Figure 1.2.

He draws attention to the fact that, when we want to learn from something that has already happened to us, we need to recall our observations of the event and then reflect on those observations in some way. We do this through reflective processes that ask us to recall and describe the experience, then

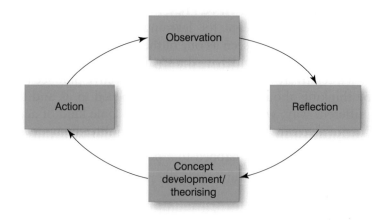

Figure 1.2   Kolb's experiential learning cycle (1984)

analyze it so that, at the end, we form some ideas or theories about it. As a result of these reflections we come to a deeper understanding of what has happened and therefore develop our own theories or concepts about it. In other words, we **transform** our understanding of that experience and see it differently. Once we have these ideas in our heads, Kolb suggests that we think about some action as a result and that this possible course of action is seen as our 'learning'. This will then inform any action that we take as a result of the experience.

The cyclical nature of reflective practice is the key to moving forward as practitioners, in that we rarely stop at just the one cycle. If we complete the first cycle, i.e. we *consciously* take action as a result of the reflective processes we have undertaken, then the next time we have that experience, or one similar to it, we will encounter it in a different way. Thus, the experience itself has been transformed, making it into a different experience. So, if we go through the cycle again, we are building our knowledge and understanding of it each time. This can be seen as a continual spiral incorporating several reflective cycles, as shown in Figure 1.3.

> **Transform**
> To change the nature, condition or function of something

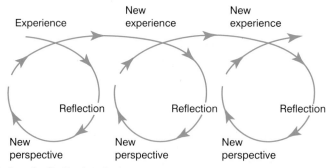

Figure 1.3   Cycles of reflective learning

Not only are we adding to our learning each time we go through a reflective cycle, we are building our underpinning knowledge base. So these successive cycles can be seen as an ever-growing spiral of knowledge development, as illustrated in Figure 1.4.

Figure 1.4   A spiral of knowledge development

In many ways this resembles a tornado; as experiences and the resultant learning grow, they 'suck up' other things as well, so that links are made to previous knowledge and experience. This process helps us to make sense of what happens to us and ever-widens our perspectives. In this way, you will start to make links between the theoretical knowledge gained in educational settings and the practice experiences you meet in the working environment.

Reflective learning, then, is not simply a matter of thinking about something that has already happened as a retrospective activity. It can also be seen as a predictive activity. It can be a strategy for planning our learning for the future, on the basis of what we already know and on what we can anticipate we will need to know. Guiding the whole reflective process is the desire to come to a deeper understanding about something that has happened to us and to maximize the learning that can result from it. Consequently, we need to be open to different ways of looking at our experiences in order to develop as practitioners, and to develop what can be called a 'reflective attitude'.

You need to understand the basics to learn,
like a wall needs a solid foundation.

KEY POINTS

- Reflective practice is a strategy that we can use to learn from our practice
- It consists of the ERA cycle (experience, reflection, action)
- It enables us to build a knowledge base from our experiences

WHY DO WE REFLECT?

We engage in reflective activity for a number of reasons. Perhaps the most basic is the need for us to develop strategies for survival throughout our lives. If we are unable to build life skills as a result of learning from our experiences, we are at risk. For instance, think of how we develop the capacity to cross a road by ourselves, and how challenging this might be for a person with an intellectual disability.

Although most of us have developed reflective strategies to ensure that we do learn as a result of what happens to us, generally we would not regard this as a fundamental way to build up our knowledge and skills. It is only when we are asked to consider the ways in which we learn best, and identify how we have learned what we know, that we start to think consciously about how we learn throughout life. The ways in which you have come to be the person you are and the ways in which you learn will be explored in Chapter 2.

KEY POINTS

The list below provides a quick summary of the purposes of reflective practice:

- To identify learning needs
- To identify new opportunities for learning
- To identify the ways in which we learn best
- To identify new courses of action
- To explore alternative ways of solving problems
- For personal development
- For professional development
- To escape routine practice
- To be aware of the consequences of our actions
- To demonstrate our competence to others
- To demonstrate our achievements to ourselves and others
- To build theory from observations
- To help us make decisions or resolve uncertainty
- To empower or emancipate ourselves as individuals

TYPES OF REFLECTION

For the purposes of this book, reflection is divided into two types – reflection-*in*-action and reflection-*on*-action. These were identified by Donald Schön (1983) as the principal ways that professionals use to conceptualize and articulate their knowledge.

Reflection-in-action

Reflection-in-action is the way that people think and theorize about practice whilst they are doing it. This is often seen as an automatic activity that occurs subconsciously in practice at an everyday level. It is thought by some people to be intuitive and an 'unconscious' process, and therefore not really a reflective activity that we use deliberately. It is often seen as the way that advanced practitioners practise. It results from a combination of their knowledge, skills and practice. This is not to say that we don't all use reflection-in-action to some degree when practising. We sift through alternatives and choose to do what we do without really being aware that we are doing it. Examples of this are when we use our interpersonal skills in a facilitative way, such as encouraging a child to take an unpleasant medicine or reacting to a casualty, who is bleeding profusely at the scene of an accident. These examples illustrate how we are able, almost instantaneously, to select from a range of options we have encountered from our own experience or draw on theoretical knowledge and select the most appropriate way of dealing with the situation in front of us.

Reflection-on-action

Reflection-on-action involves consciously exploring an experience and thinking about your practice after it has occurred, discovering the knowledge used in that situation. It occurs through analysis, interpretation and the recombination of information about the experience so that new perspectives are formed about what has happened. This usually occurs retrospectively and away from the scene of practice. It assumes that practice is underpinned by knowledge and is thus a cognitive process. Reflection-on-action can therefore be seen as an *active* process of transforming experience into knowledge and involves much more than simply thinking about and describing practice in order to understand it. Reflection-on-action also helps us to identify our knowledge gaps, and to identify missing pieces of theory or practice that we need to find, to ensure that we have a sound evidence base on which to make decisions and base our future practice. Examples of this may be:

Cognitive
Involving thoughtful, conscious understanding

- a student nurse sitting down with a staff nurse to talk through the cardiac arrest procedure after she has witnessed it
- a case discussion between a student physiotherapist and clinical supervisor that involves reviewing the student's work with their patient case load and planning resultant action.

Reflection-on-action will be focussed on throughout this book in considering the conscious development of strategies for reflective practice as learning from and for practice. However, Rolfe and colleagues (2011) explore the concept of reflection-in-action further in relation to the ways that advanced practitioners may be using reflective strategies as part of their everyday practice.

LEVELS OF REFLECTION

Goodman (1984) suggests that there are three levels of reflection that a reflective practitioner may achieve. These are shown in Table 1.1.

Table 1.1   Goodman's levels of reflection (1984)
1st level **Reflection to reach given objectives** – criteria for reflection are limited to technocratic issues of efficiency, effectiveness and accountability
2nd level **Reflection on the relationship between principles and practice** – there is an assessment of the implications and consequences of actions and beliefs as well as the underlying rationale for practice
3rd level **Reflection which besides the above incorporates ethical and political concerns** – issues of justice and emancipation enter the deliberations over the value of professional goals and practice and the practitioner makes links between the setting of everyday practice and broader social structure and forces.

As a student you will be expected to work your way up through these gradually, beginning with the first level, which is mainly descriptive. As you move through your course, becoming more familiar with the strategies used in reflective practice and more comfortable with your skills and knowledge, you will also be expected to start using the second and third levels. These will help you to explore the complex incidents and situations that you encounter in practice by drawing on theoretical perspectives and evidence – the personal and professional aspects and the ethical and political issues that are a feature of the society in which we live.

Goodman's levels are explored further, and illustrated, in Chapter 3.

KEY POINTS

● Reflection can be used for a number of different purposes

● There are two types of reflection – reflection-in-action and reflection-on-action

● Goodman identified three levels of reflection

● Reflective practice is more than simply a retrospective look at what we do, it is about understanding our actions, our knowledge base and existing skills, recognizing gaps in these and identifying what more we need to do to remedy deficits

EXPERIENCE-REFLECTION-ACTION

It is worth taking more time here to establish what we mean by the three ERA components. Remember, ERA stands for 'experience–reflection–action'. These form the foundation on which you will build your knowledge and skills for reflective practice and it is therefore important that you understand their principles. All strategies for reflection use these three components in different ways and use different words to describe them – but the underlying principles remain the same.

The nature of experience

What is experience?

There are several different ways that we can look at the idea of experience. First, we might say 'I had an exciting experience the other day'. Used in this way, the word 'experience' means something that has happened to us that we are aware of and can describe. For instance, this might have been a visit to a particular place or a meeting with someone. We might refer to this as 'an' experience and are using the word as a noun to mean something in itself. This suggests that we ourselves have taken part in the experience and therefore have first-hand knowledge of it.

Second, we may say 'She has a lot of experience in counselling distressed teenagers', in which case we are referring to an accumulation of knowledge and skill built up over time in a particular area. This means the totality of the experiences a person has had.

Finally, we might say 'I experienced something strange yesterday', in which case we are using the word as a verb, something that we 'do' or have done. In this sense, 'to experience something' means that we have done it or gone through it.

Experience can be classified into different types such as: physical, mental, emotional, spiritual, religious, social, virtual and subjective. The three that have most relevance when considering reflective practice are mental, emotional and subjective experiences. Mental experiences involve an aspect of the intellect and consciousness, i.e. awareness, and are experienced as combinations of thought, perception, memory, emotion, will and imagination, and include all unconscious processes as well. Emotional experiences relate to how we feel about something, and our capacity for empathy. Finally, experiences are recognized as being subjective – individual perceptions build our own notions of reality, based on our interaction with our environment. No-one else will ever experience something in the way you do, even if they have been beside you and witnessed the same thing happening.

Experience as a general concept results in 'know-how' or 'on-the-job' training rather than book learning. An important distinction for reflective practice is made in that experience is seen as something very practical. It is the 'doing' or 'feeling' of something rather than any thoughts about it.

KEY POINTS

This is the definition of experience used throughout the book. So, in summary, an experience may be:

● Something that has happened to you

● The *accumulation of knowledge and skills* over time, or

● The *processes* that you go though when you do something

Over to you

It's worth getting your understanding of experience really clear in your mind. If you are still wondering exactly what is being talked about as the basis for your reflective activity, search a few dictionary definitions, or look at some of the Further Reading suggestions at the end of this chapter to broaden your understanding of the concept.

So the first-hand experiences that we have as the basis for learning within practice settings are fundamental to the concept of reflective practice.

When experiences are talked about, in this book, they mean anything that might have happened to you in the past. This does not necessarily have to be related to your professional field. In fact, very often we learn a great deal about ourselves by exploring how we act in just one setting, recognizing the ways we do this and deliberately transferring that strategy to unfamiliar situations. This book will be using many of your past experiences in this way later, to help you recognize the ways you deal with the different things thrown at you in life. From these exercises you will come to understand how you react in different circumstances and the strategies you already have for coping with the world. You will also be presented with other experiences to help you to develop further in your professional roles.

However, we can go through the whole of our lives having experiences and not necessarily learning from them or, at least, not being aware that we have learned from them. Fundamental to the concept of reflective practice is that we *consciously* or *knowingly* consider our experiences in order to draw out our learning. Hence, learning from experience becomes a deliberate act, rather than it happening by accident.

Reflective activity

Make two lists of the things that you have done over the past week. On one side of the page, write down ten things that you would consider as routine or regular experiences. In this list might be things like 'catching the bus to university'; 'collecting the children from school'; 'doing the weekly shopping'. Your second list will be ten things that have been different from your usual experiences. These will probably stick out more in your mind because of this – for instance, you may have booked a holiday, been to a party, received a piece of work back from a tutor or learned a new skill at work.

Select one of the experiences in your first list, and think about how you did it. Ask yourself the following questions:

- What did I do?

- Why did I do it the way I did?

- What other ways could I have done it?

- How did I know to do it the way I did?

- What had I learned from doing it previously that means that I did it the way I did?

Now repeat this using an experience from your second list, answering these extra questions as well:

- What experience, or previous learning, have I drawn on to inform this experience?

- What new learning has occurred?

- What have I learned that I will be able to use in the future?

How often do you take time to sit down and consider your everyday experiences and think about how it is that you come to do as you do? In fact, how often do we really know what it is that we do? We tend to go through most of our days in a routine way that enables us to pack all the things that we need to do into our time, often without thinking about them. In fact, if we did think about them, there's a chance that we'd never get anything done at all! We'd be slowed up by consciously having to think about everything we do. It is even possible that we would not be as efficient at what we do, simply because we are thinking about it. For instance, people who drive a car regularly do not think about the mechanics of driving; they do it automatically. They concentrate on the driving conditions and respond to the circumstances they are in. If they were thinking about every gear change or clutch depression, it is likely that they would drive dangerously because their full attention would not be on the road. It is also probable that the quality of their driving would deteriorate because cognitive processes were interfering with what had become instinctive practice. An illustration of this is the insecurity that can arise when we have to drive in a country that uses the other side of the road or where familiar road layouts change, such as at road works, and we are suddenly jolted into a consciousness that something is different and we need to take notice.

In looking back at your answers to the exercise, can you identify elements of this happening to you in the first example that you used? How much of your efficiency is due to the fact that the way you do something has become ingrained; so much so that you are unaware of how you are doing it? Yet, at one time, you were not this efficient. You have built the ability up through repetition and things have become second nature. It does not even occur to you to do things differently unless you consciously make a decision to think of alternatives. This often happens as a result of watching someone else do the same thing, but in a different way from ourselves. For instance, you might watch the way another person does a task and think 'What are they doing it like that for? It's much easier the way I do it!', or perhaps the opposite, that they seem to achieve a better or quicker result than you. As a result, you might decide to change the way that you do the task yourself.

In the second example that you used, you may have found that you were more conscious of what you were doing at the time you were doing it, and therefore found it easier to answer the questions. It is in unfamiliar situations, or those that occur less frequently, that we tend to think consciously about what we are doing. Perhaps we then refer to the rules that we have learned, or drag explanations out from our subconscious in order to make decisions and take action – or to justify that action. For instance, if you are booking a holiday, you will be actively drawing on your previous experiences in order to make decisions about the future – things, such as whether to use a travel agent or price comparison websites; the type of place you want to go and the type of accommodation that will suit your needs; and the amount of money that you have to spend. Other things that will occur to you may involve checking your passport, booking your dog into kennels and ordering a taxi to take you to the airport. Other people focus on preparing the house so that it is secure, and hiding valuables.

None of these considerations happen either automatically or by accident. They come into your mind as a result of thoughtful processes that draw on your previous experiences of booking a holiday. You draw on experiences with similar features that enable you to apply what you have learned from one situation to another. It is this deliberate activity of using reflective processes to explore our experiences that enables us to identify, acknowledge and value our experiential learning. We need to know more about these reflective processes in order to use them effectively to learn from our experiences.

KEY POINTS

- Everything that happens to us can be seen as an experience that can be reflected on and learned from
- We can transfer our learning from one experience into others
- We need to consciously use our experiences as the starting point of our learning

WHAT ARE REFLECTIVE PROCESSES?

Reflective processes help us to see the world in alternative ways by enabling us to focus on different aspects of our experiences. By reflective processes we mean the stages of thoughtful activity we go through when we consciously decide to explore an experience. There are many ways in which we can reflect, and a variety of strategies for doing this are discussed in Chapter 3. In this section, however, the basic ideas behind using a structure for reflecting that run throughout all the strategies you will meet later are outlined, whether you are reflecting by yourself or with other people.

The fundamental stages of the reflective processes are:

- Stage 1: Selecting a critical incident to reflect on
- Stage 2: Observing and describing the experience
- Stage 3: Analyzing the experience
- Stage 4: Interpreting the experience
- Stage 5: Exploring alternatives
- Stage 6: Framing action

Stage 1: Selecting a critical incident to reflect on

The critical incident

As seen in the previous section, any experience we have can be used as a focus for reflection. However, what we choose to reflect on needs to have some significance for us, in terms of what we are trying to achieve or the purpose it is going to serve. When reflecting for learning as part of a course, you need to identify events that will contribute to your learning as a developing practitioner; therefore these events need to be significant in some way. Throughout this book, these events are referred to as critical incidents.

> **Critical incident**
> Event that stands out in your mind and contributes directly to development as a practitioner

Paul and critical incidents

Paul found thousands of references to reflective practice in his Google search. He now understands that it is about not only learning from experience, but about using this learning in future practice. However, he is still confused about what is meant by a 'critical incident'. As a student paramedic, understands the word 'critical' to mean life-threatening or very serious. Surely though, he won't be expected to identify this kind of 'critical' incident every day, or even throughout his practice? He realizes that it is important to check out concepts or definitions of words that are familiar or seem to have a common meaning, before taking them for granted.

The term 'critical incident' was first coined in 1954 by John Flanagan, a psychologist working with the US Air Force. He defined it in the following way:

> " *By an incident is meant any observable human activity that is sufficiently complete in itself to permit inferences and predictions to be made about the person performing the act. To be critical, an incident must occur in a situation where the purpose or intent of the act seems fairly clear to the observer and where its consequences are sufficiently definite to leave little doubt concerning its effects.*
>
> *Flanagan 1954, p. 327*

To simplify this: critical incidents can be seen as episodes of experience that have particular meaning to the observer, practitioner or any other person taking part in them. They may be positive or negative experiences and must be suitable for being described in a concise way. Critical incidents are usually seen as something that has already happened to us but in this book the definition is broadened out in terms of anticipating the future as well. While you are not expected to have a crystal ball, as a student there is a certain degree of predictability about the experiences you will have during your course. By reflecting on what is coming up, in terms of placements in the working environment or university work, you can anticipate your learning needs and plan to use your time more effectively. Similarly, you will have been given learning outcomes for your course, and all disciplines will have practical skills or competencies to be achieved before you can be licensed to practise your profession. So, in terms of the subject matter for reflective practice and learning, thinking about what you need to achieve is as significant as thinking about any of the experiences you have already had.

When a critical incident is significant, it sticks in our minds for a number of reasons. These may be because it made us feel good or valued, or that we felt we were doing a good job or had achieved success at something. It may also be because it made us feel angry or dejected or devalued in some way. We might also feel that negative consequences were our fault, or a result of actions we took that were somehow wrong, or that we made a mistake that has resulted in someone suffering. Other examples might be a comment you made to someone that was taken in a different way from the one in which it was meant, and a row exploded, or that you hear that someone is saying things about you that you think are unfair or untrue. Unfortunately, the term 'critical incident' has often been misunderstood within the context of reflective practice. Part of the reason for this lies in the fact that we are working in health care professions, where the word 'critical' is often used to mean 'serious'. If we go back to Flanagan's definition, though, we can see that this was not the original intention. Flanagan meant 'critical' to mean something important or stands out in some way, and this is the way in which the term will be used in this book.

Of course, when you think about it logically, we tend to build on success. In the past many of us unconsciously repeated actions and ways of working that had previously been successful and avoided ones that had not. The overt use of reflective processes, and critical reflection at that, is to enable us to learn deliberately from our experiences and to identify action that can be taken in the future.

Sources for reflection can therefore come from any experience we have had, and we can learn from things that have gone well just as effectively as from negative experiences. In fact, the reason that we tend to dwell on things that go wrong is that for most of the time everything in our lives goes well, and we take this for granted!

Reflective activity

Think back over the previous week and list all the things that have happened to you that you felt didn't turn out as you wanted them to.

Now make a list of everything that went successfully. How long is the second list in comparison to the first one?

We don't tend to give ourselves much credit for everyday things that go right – getting to university on time, for instance, or ensuring that there is enough bread and milk in the house for breakfast. But, if these things don't happen, we are likely to remember and take steps to prevent the situation from occurring again. It is a natural instinct to avoid situations that will cause us stress and make us feel uncomfortable. We learn to take things that go right in our stride and not to focus on them; as a result we do not give ourselves credit for our part in them. Hence, when something does go wrong, whether it is our fault or not, we tend to blame ourselves and feel guilty and uncomfortable. It is a natural drive to want to avoid these stressful feelings, so we reflect on what has happened in order to learn from the experience and change our behaviour.

 Case study

Paul begins reflective practice

Paul thinks he's got it! He was really worried to start with that he wouldn't be able to think of any experiences important enough to be used as the basis for his learning. After all, he is just a beginner! But, he's realized that it makes sense to try to identify things from the past that have happened and explore them in some way to attempt to understand his own ways of dealing with incidents and learn for the future. He's had a go at thinking about how he reacts to stressful situations, remembering when his friend Jack had the motorbike accident, and considers himself to be calm under pressure – a good start for a paramedic!

The focus for reflective activity has widened as reflective processes have developed into mainstream techniques for learning in courses, and apply to all the outcomes that need to be achieved by students. Hence, reflective processes are now used not only to learn from things that have already happened but also to plan learning experiences to fulfil identified needs on the basis of the experiences we have already had. Some universities are now using reflective practice as the main strategy for learning in their health practitioner educational courses, incorporating within it all other learning and teaching strategies.

We can see, therefore, that the selection of experiences has become important in ensuring that students are able to maximize the learning they achieve. In addition to identifying an experience solely for reasons of what you can learn from it, there are other issues to take into account.

The other people involved

As a student health care practitioner, it is unlikely that you will be working in isolation. Hence, in the majority of experiences other people will be involved, ranging from the patients you are caring for, their relatives and other carers, to your fellow students and colleagues, supervisors, other practitioners and educational staff.

You may need to consider all the other people involved, both as part of the experience itself and in the reflective activity.

The type of event involving other people you choose to reflect on will depend on whether your reflective activity is going to be shared with other people. Will others be involved in exploring the case with you or reading a reflective account of it? If you are choosing the event solely for your own purposes, and the results of your reflections will be kept private, you do not have to worry about any far-reaching consequences of what you are doing. However, if the event is to be shared with others you need to take into account several issues. These are covered in more detail in Chapter 6 and are simply summarized here as markers.

When focusing on events involving other people you need to think about:

- The effect this might have on the other people involved
- Gaining consent from the others involved
- The status of any written records you might make
- Confidentiality and protecting others.

When considering reflecting with others in a professional context, think about:

- The contextual implications of discussing things that have happened
- Choosing what to tell and considering the implications of this
- Working within professional codes of conduct and discussing the implications of this
- The consequences of disclosure
- Misconduct/malpractice/negligence
- Understanding the responsibilities of others within their professional role.

Establishing the purpose of your reflective activity

Finally, the reasons why you are reflecting will affect what it is that you choose to reflect on, and several of these were outlined on p. 6. Establishing the purpose of your reflection will help you to select from the experiences available and match up the experience with the outcome.

KEY POINTS

- Experiences for reflection can come from a multitude of sources, such as:

  - Any part of your life

  - Things that have gone well

  - Things that make you happy

  - Things that you feel uncomfortable about

  - Things that have made you sad

  - Things that have gone wrong

  - Observations that other people have made about you

  - Your relationships with others

- Selecting an experience to reflect on depends on:

  - The purpose of your reflection, i.e. why you are doing it

  - Who else may be part of the experience or incident, e.g. patients, carers, other professional staff

  - Who else may be part of the reflective process, i.e. talking or reading about your experiences

  - The possible consequences

- All experiences can be seen as *critical incidents* because they were important to us and stick in our mind in some way, contributing to our professional development

- When choosing an incident to reflect on it is important to consider the roles that other people played in it

- It is important to identify the purpose of reflecting on the incident chosen

Stage 2: Observing and describing the experience

The purpose of this stage of the reflective process is to produce as full a description of your experience as possible. It is helpful, especially when you are beginning reflective practice, to use a framework of key questions to structure the description of your experiences. These help you to focus on the essential structure of what happened and ensure that you consider all aspects of it. Some of these frameworks are explored and illustrated in Chapter 3.

A useful *aide memoire* for guiding this and the next two stages of the ERA cycle is what has come to be known as the six wise men.

These are the words that start the questions that you will be asking, and are worth committing to memory to help you start reflective practice. They are:

- Who
- What
- Where
- When
- Why
- How

These are often used for training journalists to take down the key elements of a story they are reporting on, so they don't miss anything out. The first four will be used in the descriptive phase, whereas you will use the 'why' and 'how' questions in the analytical and interpretive phases as you come to understand more deeply what has happened. They do not necessarily need to be used in this order, however. As you become more familiar with strategies for reflective practice you will find that you re-order the ways in which you use the cue questions to suit the experience you are reflecting on and the purpose you want it to achieve.

This will provide the basic record of the event and the data you use as raw material for the later stages. You can either do this verbally or create a written record.

To write or not to write?

You have the choice of writing, or not writing, the description of your experiences. Written reflection has a different character to contemplative or verbal reflection, and detailed consideration is given to this in Chapter 5. In this you will explore the features of written reflection by looking at:

- The reason why we write
- How we can use writing to help order our thoughts
- The purpose of creating a permanent record
- How we can be creative through writing
- Using writing to develop our analytical skills
- Using writing to develop our critical thinking
- Using writing to develop new understandings and knowledge
- Using writing to show that we understand
- Writing in the first person (i.e. writing 'I went', 'I felt')

Do remember that your memory of an event will change over time, as our minds select what they consider to be the most significant parts of the experience to suit their purpose at any given time. For instance, close to a traumatic event, you will concentrate on your emotional reactions, as these enable you to deal with the situation and to take action to prevent yourself from being harmed. Therefore, you are likely to focus on the cause of your distress and attempt to justify your reactions and feelings. Later, however, when you are feeling safer, your mind will allow you to think more widely and perhaps more rationally, about the situation, and therefore your reflections will be different. Written records bring benefits here, in that they allow you to record and then revisit your records as many times as you want after the events. This is something that reflecting verbally may not offer you: it may be restricted to a particular occasion and person that might not be available at a later date. Verbal reflection also takes place at a particular time, whether close to the event or at some other stage. Again, this brings its own benefits and drawbacks, and these are considered in Chapter 5.

KEY POINTS

- The purpose of the description is to get as full a picture of what happened as possible
- The 'six wise men' can be used as cue questions: these are who, what, where, when, why, how
- Writing an incident down provides a different perspective to thoughtful or spoken reflection

Stage 3: Analyzing the experience

At this stage in the process, you will be starting to take some steps back from your experience and attempting to treat it more objectively as a source of data to be broken down into its constituent parts. Here you start to ask the 'why' type of question as you explore the reasons behind what has happened. Now you are moving beyond the superficial elements of the first four key questions and it is here that you will draw conclusions from what you have recorded about the experience. As you progress through your course, and your academic career, you will increasingly be expected to reflect more deeply and with more insight, so that you achieve the key skills for the level at which you are studying. The skills of analysis are perhaps the first of these to be developed, as you move from the descriptive phases.

Analysis simply means to break things down into their constituent parts. For example, if you send a blood sample to a laboratory for 'analysis', what you get reported back are the proportions of its constituents. However, we expect analysis to go a little further than this, in terms of making some sort of judgement on the basis of this information. A laboratory report will, for instance, highlight where levels are within normal limits or fall outside of them. So, at this stage in our reflective processes, we will be expecting you to draw some preliminary conclusions as to the result of your analysis, such as 'What felt right about this experience and why?', or 'What actions caused this to go wrong, and why was this?'

> **Analysis**
> Breaking things down and forming preliminary conclusions

When you first start reflective practice as part of your professional education, this is the stage at which you will probably stop. You will have begun to develop insight into the experiences you are exploring and to reach some conclusions about the part you played in them. This conscious awareness is crucial to the learning process, as we can use it to determine our future action. However, as you progress through your course, you will be expected to progress further through the levels of reflection (discussed in Chapter 3).

It is also at this stage that you may start to feel some discomfort about reflective practice as a strategy for learning. It may bring back memories of how you felt at the time or, alternatively, you may start to realize that what happened was a direct result of your part in the incident – what you did, how you acted, the choices you made. This is an inevitable part of using your own experiences to learn and a consequence of deliberately deciding to use these experiences as a source of learning. However, to some extent this is a very mature way of learning. We need to be willing to revisit our own actions, and we need to have some insight into ourselves. We also need to be able to accept responsibility for our own actions and the choices we make. For many students starting out on this path will be difficult, and that is why you will be asked to build reflective skills and strategies gradually. Part of this is to help you with your own self-development as you grow through your course. A professional, who is expected to develop as an independent practitioner, needs not only the knowledge and practical skills of their profession but also the insight and acceptance of their own actions that marks them as a responsible and safe practitioner. It is through the use of reflective practice, and developing the skills gradually and in a safe environment with the help of others, that you will add these skills to the 'kitbag' of tools that you use in your practice.

So, at this stage in the process, you may come to conclusions that you don't like very much or you feel reflect badly on you. However, this is not something to be anxious about provided that you remember:

1 what the purpose of exploring the situation was
2 what you hope to get out of it in terms of learning for the future.

KEY POINTS

- Analyzing means 'breaking experiences down and coming to some preliminary conclusions about them'
- You may begin to see the experience in a different way at this stage

Stage 4: Interpreting the experience

During this stage you will develop a deeper understanding of the experience by exploring the different parts of it further. In the last stage you broke your experience down under different headings, such as 'What did I do and why?'

or 'What did the other person do and why?' Here we want you to start thinking behind all these questions so that you understand a bit more about why things happened in the way that they did. You may choose to concentrate on just one or two of the features here and deal with them in detail. What you will end up with at this stage of the process is an *explanation*. This will enable you to move to the next phase of exploring alternatives, both interpreting the experience differently and seeing it in a different way.

Again, it is at this stage that you might find the process uncomfortable. Awkward questions may start popping into your head that you really don't want to think about. Or you may find that the incident dominates your thoughts when you are not deliberately reflecting on it. Don't worry! This is entirely natural and is part of the process of learning to reflect. As you become more skilled in the process you will be able to train yourself to limit your reflective activity to specific times that you set aside for it – maybe with other people or to compile a reflective journal for instance. At this stage in the process, though, try to focus on the future – think about the resolution of the process. The final two stages will bring you back to the top of the reflective cycle and will help you to move away from the experience as it was, into perceptions of the experience that you haven't thought about; and what action you need to take as a result. These final stages are the 'feel good' stages, where you can resolve a situation and decide to *deliberately* do something as a result of your explorations.

KEY POINTS

- Interpretation involves considering your experiences in the light of other knowledge
- This will provide you with an explanation of the experience

Stage 5: Exploring alternatives

At this stage you will be thinking about alternatives to the ways in which you saw your experience initially. This is very challenging, in that it is asking you to look at different ways of understanding the experience to the way that you have described. Imagine looking at your experience as if you are not you at all! You will be trying to step out of your skin and see the whole experience from different viewpoints. To do this by yourself is quite difficult, so, initially, you will meet various different ways of reflecting, and be introduced to them in a variety of ways and in many settings – both academic and in the practice environment. You will also be encouraged to reflect with different people, for example, colleagues, practice supervisors, other professional practitioners and academic advisors. From this you will build up a bank of both differing ways of reflecting and differing viewpoints from which to consider your experiences. The benefit of working within a multi-professional environment is that we are always meeting others whose background provides them with different ways of seeing things, interpreting and explaining them. This enables us, in turn, to question our 'taken-for-granted' views and explorations of the world. Other people can help us when we cannot see a different way of doing something and helps us to move beyond our personal involvement in an event and see it more objectively.

One way to understand the concept of viewing experiences from alternative perspectives, is to think of the way that the world appears if we put on different types of spectacles. Try to imagine how the world would look if we altered the types of spectacles that we wear (think of sun glasses if you don't wear spectacles to correct your vision). For instance, if you smeared the lenses with grease, you would not have the clarity of view that you normally have, and everything would be out of focus. You would have to turn to your other senses, and your experience, to fill the gaps in the knowledge you use to make sense of what you are seeing. Another example is the way in which our perceptions change when it is dark – some things are hidden from us, we do not have the familiarity of colour and detail to help us and we have to rely on other ways of gaining information to help us to make decisions.

This is exactly what we do at this stage of the reflective process, in that we look for alternative ways of 'seeing' the experience. We have to use our other senses in order to 'see' things in a different way. We do this without thinking when we are dealing with the physical processes of trying to see in the dark. We automatically use our other senses to pick up on different cues that we don't need to use in daylight. We may even choose to focus on one or two specific elements of the experience, like putting something under a microscope and examining it in more detail.

At this stage in the reflective process, we will be consciously seeking ways of seeing the features of our experiences in a different way, for the purpose of learning more about them.

We may do this by ourselves, and use a reflective framework to help us, or we may choose to use others to reflect off, and use their perceptions to help us to see things from a different perspective.

The purpose of this stage, therefore, is to widen and deepen the experience for us by exploring other ways of 'seeing' what has occurred. Once we have done this, we can move to the final stage, which involves deciding how we can use what we have learned to identify what we need to do in the future.

KEY POINTS

- Exploring alternatives is a challenging process as it asks us to step outside of our usual ways of seeing our experiences
- This stage enables us to explore alternative ways of perceiving things and working to those we would normally use

Stage 6: Framing action

Arising from the previous stage will be several different possibilities for action that you might take. It is important here to make sure that you focus on *your* activity rather than expecting others to act for you or change themselves. This is *your* reflective learning and thus you only have responsibility for yourself – others hold their own responsibilities and make their own choices. While it may be comforting to propose courses of action for others that will make our lives easier, in reality motivation for change inevitably comes from within oneself. What we would like to see someone else do is not necessarily the right course of action for them, nor one that they would choose. Also, it will not necessarily alter the action or consequences for you in the end. How often have you said of a partner or a friend 'If only they would do what I told them to, it would all be so much simpler!'? Unfortunately, life isn't like that.

So, the focus for framing action is on things that you can do that are within your control.

Of course, if you are helping another person to reflect, perhaps in clinical supervision or in a reflective activity, then your role will be to enable them to see their own alternatives and you may be able to suggest courses of action that they themselves haven't seen. As a result you may also shift your perspective and decide to change your own ways of dealing with something.

The differences between reflective processes and reflective practice

Up to the end of this stage, what we have done is explore reflective processes, rather than necessarily reflective practice. We have not moved into the last element of reflective practice, which is to take the action that we have decided on.

At the end of the last stage, we were still operating in the realms of theoretical activity; we were talking about possibilities and what we might do. This could be, for instance, what we would do if the situation occurred again. Or it may be that we need to go to the library and get more information to add to the knowledge that underpinned how we dealt with the incident. Another possibility is that we decide we need to go and talk to someone else who is able to influence a situation that we are in. So, no action has been taken but the different courses of action have been explored.

It is important at this stage to consider not only what you might do but also the possible consequences of any course of action that you might take. In this way, a decision not to take action can be a deliberate choice, and in many ways is action! It differs from inactivity before reflection on the event because you have now thought through all aspects of the incident and consciously decided that overt action is not needed. You will, however, have a deeper understanding of the event and, perhaps more importantly, an understanding and overt acknowledgement of what you have learned about the experience.

Planning action has several features. First of all, the alternatives that you select from need to be possible in terms of:

- the scope of what you are trying to achieve
- the outcome you are trying to achieve
- how much you will need to rely on the help of other people
- the barriers you may encounter
- the resources you may need to carry the action out.

Secondly, you need to be capable of carrying out the action. You will need to think about:

- the time it will take
- having access to relevant people
- your own knowledge, skills and experiences
- your motivation to carry out the action.

Finally, you will need to think about the consequences of any action that you might be considering, in terms of:

- yourself
- your patients/clients
- your colleagues
- your mentor/supervisor
- other professional work colleagues
- academic staff
- your workplace
- your role as a student
- working within the code of professional conduct.

This may seem like a long list, and rather daunting at first. However, most of the time you will not need to consider all these aspects, and the list is here simply for you to think about when framing and planning any action. But sometimes we do omit to think about the consequences of the things that we do, and often this results in the unexpected coming at us. Hence, a cornerstone of professional practice is the ability to think through alternative courses of action in terms of the anticipated consequences for all concerned.

Once you have decided on the action that you will take from all of the possible viewpoints, you are ready to carry it out.

KEY POINTS

- Framing action enables us to consider our future actions arising from the incident and its analysis
- The reflective processes end at this stage
- Reflective practice differs from reflective processes in that we turn thoughtful and possible activity into action

TAKING ACTION

As the final phase of reflective practice, this is where you will carry out the action that you have decided upon. This can be the easiest part of being a reflective practitioner – but it can also be the hardest! This will depend of course on what it is that you have to do. It is here that you will move from the realms of the possible and probable into the real world. For instance, going to the library to research a topic to increase your knowledge is unlikely to be stressful. But other courses of action, especially where they involve confronting others or doing things that you find challenging or difficult and involve changes to your usual patterns of behaviour, will inevitably involve some anxiety or stress. This is entirely natural, and the way to manage it is to think about all the possible results of your action and plan for them in advance. As a practitioner in the future you will need to way up the levels of stress that you are able to tolerate – this is where you get the practice!

Factors you might like to consider are:

- **What you want to achieve as a result of your action.** This is where you will have reached the last stage of the reflective processes, so you should now have an idea of what your goals are in taking action. It is worth trying to describe your goal concisely as a single sentence, so that you have it clearly fixed in your mind. This also helps you to focus on the main purpose of taking action and to be single-minded in achieving your goal.

- **How you will do it.** Again, thinking through the possibilities of how you will take action helps you feel in control of the situation. You might like to plan the overall strategy that you will adopt, including:

  - **When you will do it?** We have all heard the wisdom of 'sleeping on a problem'. It is often worth waiting before carrying out our decisions so that we can put some emotional distance between ourselves and the incident. However, just as pertinent is the need to resolve issues, so a happy medium between the two needs to be achieved. Perhaps the most important factor in terms of taking action is that it is your choice and under your control. Do you remember previous incidents that someone has caught you on the 'wrong foot' by asking to talk to you about something that you weren't expecting? For instance, were you ever called to see a teacher at school, or a supervisor at work, and you didn't know what it was about?

- **Where you will do it?**
- **Who will be part of the action?**

The importance of planning

There is an old adage 'to fail to plan is to plan to fail', and this is most appropriate in many aspects of student life. For instance, if you don't ensure that you understand what you are being asked to do in your assignments, plan your research and writing time to submit on time, or plan your revision strategies for exams, you are more likely to fail than if you did those things. Students who pass all the elements of their course haven't done so by accident, they have planned, and taken action, to pass.

Similarly, when taking action as a result of your reflective activity, you can plan to be successful by thinking through all possible elements of the action that are within your control, to reduce the possibility of things going wrong.

One way of thinking about this is to recall other instances when you have decided to do something similar. Remember the sense of relief and satisfaction that you felt once you had successfully resolved the issue. For instance, how many of us have dreaded returning goods to a shop for fear of encountering aggressive shop assistants? Yet, with forethought and careful planning, knowing our rights in the circumstances and using good interpersonal skills, it is possible for both parties to achieve what they want without any problems. The relief and positive feelings that result, enable us to reflect on that experience as a learning opportunity, leading to less stress the next time a similar thing occurs. The combination of successful encounters and the building up of cognitive skills as a result, help to reduce the feelings of stress that we experience in other situations where we are worried about taking the action we need to. On the other hand, we are always likely to feel uncomfortable about not seeing things through to a conclusion, or taking the actions that we need to, as we are not experiencing closure of the incident or of the reflective cycle.

Reflective activity

Why do you do what you do?

Think back to the last time that you successfully tackled an issue you were anxious about. Reflect over the stages of what happened and what you did.

- What were the things that you did that made the incident successful?
- What from these would you use again in similar circumstances?
- How did resolving this incident make you feel?
- Did you find that after it was resolved the incident held less importance or significance for you?

Now think of an incident where you did not follow through on the course of action that you had decided was needed.

- Why did you decide not to act?
- How satisfied are you with the outcome of what happened?
- Do you find that you still think about the incident in a negative way?
- What do you think about it now?
- Is it still unfinished business?

No-one will claim that it is easy to take action to resolve difficult situations. But the rewards of doing so are many. Not least is the fact that you will be developing strategies for working in an environment that, by necessity, has to involve interactions between other people. But unresolved situations can cause stress, as we constantly think about what we did, or didn't do. They prevent us from achieving the things that we want to do because they take up our mental energy. Sometimes we just have to 'bite the bullet' and do something in order to get it out of the way, so that we can direct our energy into things that are more creative and positive.

Of course, if we do take the action as planned, we have created a new experience for ourselves, which in turn may be the focus of reflective activity. This is how the reflective cycle turns into the reflective spiral that we saw in Figure 1.3, earlier in the chapter.

KEY POINTS

- Taking action involves moving from the possible and probable into the real world
- It involves making decisions about what you will do, when, where and how you will do it
- It involves considering the roles of other people in your action
- Planning your action is more likely to result in success
- Failing to plan is planning to fail

Identifying your role as a student in the working environment

When you enter the working environment to gain experience during your practice, it is important to remember the primary reasons for you being there. These are:

- To learn from the experiences available
- To develop your competence in the practical aspects of your profession
- To acquire the professional attributes of a practitioner.

Essentially, these come down to one thing – to learn. However, you will be entering a working environment whose primary purpose is to deliver care to patients. Supporting you as a student is a supplementary role for those working there. Their priorities will revolve around patient care, and your needs will be subsumed below this. Therefore, the main person to look out for your needs is you! It is important to remember that, while you will get a great deal of help from other people, you are the only one who can ensure that you are gaining the experience that you need in order to achieve your learning outcomes. Using strategies for reflective practice will help you to do this in a conscious and planned way.

Students of health and social care professions come from a wide range of backgrounds and life experiences. Many students now enter professional education as mature students, having already gained experience in a health care environment. For these students, entering the working environment will not be as unfamiliar as for those students who are starting their courses straight from school or with little work experience. However, it is important to remember that everyone is an individual who already has life experiences that will stand them in good stead for their course. While mature students may envy the academic skills of students who have studied more recently, those with less or no clinical experience may be considerably in awe of those who have earned a place on the course as a result of years of practical experience. It is important to remember that all students on a course are there to achieve competency in all areas of practice that will enable them to gain a professional qualification. All students enter the course having been selected because they have a profile of attributes, combining academic qualifications, a potential to achieve these, practical experience and the appropriate attitudes and values for health care professions. These profiles are different for all students, providing a wealth of experiences and qualities that can be used as a resource for supporting and learning from each other.

All students bring different strengths to their course; you can support and learn from each other.

One of these will be your own attitude towards learning, and your willingness to be open to new experiences, to put yourself in unfamiliar situations and learn from them. However much previous working experience you have, there is always more that can be learned. One of the key skills that you will need to develop as early as possible is to recognize and use learning opportunities in the working environment. These are explored in more detail in Chapter 4.

KEY POINTS

- Your primary purpose in the working environment is to learn from the experiences available
- We can use these to build on our previous experiences
- It is important to recognize learning opportunities in all environments where you have placements

CONCLUSIONS

In this chapter you have been introduced to the features of reflective practice so that you have a basic understanding to carry you through to the rest of the book. Especially important is becoming familiar with the stages of the ERA cycle through which reflective practice occurs. These stages, and the processes within them, are the key to your development as a reflective practitioner. The rest of the book develops each of the aspects that you have met in this chapter to help you acquire the skills and attributes of reflective practice by showing you how to do it.

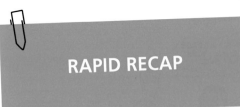

RAPID RECAP

Check your progress so far by working through each of the following questions.

1 What is the ERA cycle of reflective practice?

2 What are Schön's two types of reflection?

3 What is the difference between the reflective processes and reflective practice?

4 What are the stages in the reflective processes?

5 What is meant by the term 'critical incident'?

If you have difficulty with more than one of the questions, read through the section again to refresh your understanding before moving on.

REFERENCES

Dewey, J. (1938) *Experience and Education.* Macmillan, New York.

Flanagan, J. (1954) The Critical Incident Technique. *Psychological Bulletin*, **51**, 327–358.

Goodman, J. (1984) Reflection and teacher education: a case study and theoretical analysis. *Interchange*, **15**, 9–26.

Kolb, D. (1984) *Experiential Learning as the Science of Learning and Development.* Prentice Hall, Englewood Cliffs, NJ.

Rolfe, G., Jasper, M. and Freshwater, D. (2011) *Critical Reflection in Practice: generating knowledge for care. (2nd edition).* Palgrave, Basingstoke.

Schön, D. (1983) *The Reflective Practitioner: How professionals think in action.* Temple Smith, London.

FURTHER READING

There are both general books on reflective practice, as well as different disciplinary interpretations and ways in which they use reflection as part of their practice. Some texts have developed over time, as professions explored the ways in which reflective practice has become embedded within the ways they both learn and practice their professions. For pre-registration understanding and key reflective skills it may be worth accessing some of the following books:

Susan Lillyman and Pauline Merrix 2012 *Nursing and Health Survival Guide; Portfolios and Reflective Practice.* Pearson

Beverley Taylor 2010 *Reflective Practice for Health Care Professionals: a practical guide.* 3rd edition. Open University Press, Maidenhead

Chris Bulman and Sue Shutz 2008 *Reflective Practice in Nursing* 4th edition. Blackwell Publishing, Oxford

Lioba Howatson-Jones 2010 *Reflective Practice in Nursing (Transforming Nursing Practice).* Learning Matters, Exeter

Sue Thompson and Neil Thompson 2008 *The Critically Reflective Practitioner.* Palgrave Macmillan, Basingstoke

Sofie Bager-Charleson 2010 *Reflective Practice in Counselling and Psychotherapy.* Learning Matters, Exeter.

CHAPTER 2

KNOWING OURSELVES

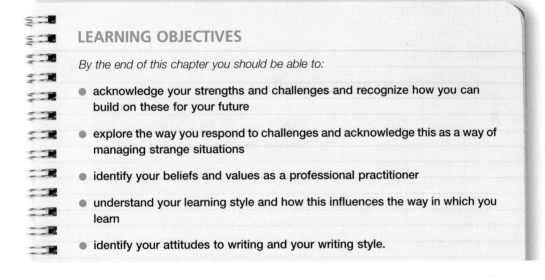

LEARNING OBJECTIVES

By the end of this chapter you should be able to:

● acknowledge your strengths and challenges and recognize how you can build on these for your future

● explore the way you respond to challenges and acknowledge this as a way of managing strange situations

● identify your beliefs and values as a professional practitioner

● understand your learning style and how this influences the way in which you learn

● identify your attitudes to writing and your writing style.

Reflective practice takes its starting point from our experiences and assumes that we can learn from them for our future. Therefore, the first place that we need to start in terms of our own reflective practice is by understanding ourselves. By knowing where we are starting from we can plan to build on our previous knowledge, understanding and skill as the foundations for our learning and development as professional practitioners. The purpose of this chapter is to lead you in recognizing and exploring your previous experiences, so that you can actively use these in planning to succeed on your course. These can also be seen as the strategies that you use in your professional practice as you utilize them for learning and managing challenges. This chapter takes your past experiences, characteristics, attitudes and approaches to life as a starting point to help you develop more understanding about yourself as a learner as well as gaining basic reflective skills so you can succeed on your course.

RECOGNIZING OUR STRENGTHS AND WEAKNESSES

How often have you sat down in the past and really thought about what you are good at? How often do we draw attention to what we consider to be our failings, without acknowledging our strengths? Yet, crucial to being able to act as a professional practitioner is, an understanding of our skills and abilities and an awareness of where the limits of these lie.

One of the ways that we can do this is to use a SWOB analysis to look analytically at ourselves. This involves thinking deeply to identify Strengths and Weaknesses. After this you broaden out into identifying what Opportunities are available to you, and what the Barriers might be in using these to achieve your aims. Key cue questions can be used to help you reflect on these four elements.

Reflective activity

| Strengths | Weaknesses |
| Opportunities | Barriers |

SWOB analysis grid

Use the grid to complete your own SWOB analysis

Start with identifying your strengths. Although you are doing this in your capacity as a health care student, do not limit what you write to simply what you think is appropriate to this role. Try to incorporate elements of all aspects of your experience such as your family life, your previous jobs, your educational experiences and any leisure time activities and interests that you have. Go behind these to identify the skills and experiences, the knowledge and understanding, that has resulted in you being the person that you are today. Some of the elements you might like to consider are:

- What are you good at?
- What is it about yourself that you are happy with?
- How do you get on with other people?
- What approaches do you take to life?
- What have you achieved so far in your life – what does this tell you about your strengths?
- What experiences have you had that provide a foundation for your course?

When thinking about your weaknesses, the purpose is not to find fault or blame yourself for anything. Instead, you will be making an honest assessment of where you feel you have room for improvement. So, initially, list all the things you can think of, whether you think they are under your control or not. Some cue questions might be:

- What would I like to change about myself?
- What things have not been successful?
- What things have I not achieved that I wanted to by now?
- What disappointments have I had that affect the ways I think about the future?

When you come to the Opportunities section try to build on what you have already identified as your strengths. For instance, if you have written 'I am good at working to deadlines' think how this can be used within your course over the next few years. Other cue questions might be:

- What is available within the course to help me?
- Who can help me?
- What support do I have that will help me?

In identifying the Barriers to your success, you might reflect on what the weaknesses you have identified tell you about yourself. How might you put up your own obstacles to success simply through the ways that you approach life? In fact, these might then become opportunities for your own development and change in the future and you may decide to move them. For instance, you may have young children who have calls on your time and therefore see this as a barrier to having as much time for study as you would wish. In fact, we all have limitations on our time for one reason or another. Having to apportion your time in various ways makes you think about the most effective ways of using it. So, you may decide that you will set aside specific time during the day that you can use for studying, and set boundaries to this. This would have the added effect of training your children so that they realize you need time to yourself and are not always at their beck and call.

Using a structure for reflection like this, provides us with new ways of looking at things. It is rare in everyday life to be able to consider what makes us the person we are. We tend to be so busy simply getting through the day that we take for granted who and what we are. The case study below presents Jaz's SWOB analysis.

 Case study

Jaz

Jaz has just started a four year, full-time course for a dual qualification as a Social Worker and Registered Nurse for People with Learning Disabilities. She is a mature student of Caribbean background living in London, aged 36, a single mother with two teen-aged sons, and an elderly father living with her. She has spent the last ten years in youth and community work support roles, gaining a variety of experience in social work and social care settings. She decided that she would like to gain professional qualifications so went to her local college part-time to study an access course which gained her admission to the University where mature students with work experience are particularly welcomed.

Jaz's SWOB analysis

Strengths

I have had ten years, experience as a care worker in social care, youth work and a residential home for young people with severe learning disabilities

I understand the challenges of working with people with communication problems

I have good practical skills

I am not afraid of hard work

I am highly motivated and determined to succeed

I am good at communicating with people

I am very patient with other people

I am an optimist – nothing much gets me down

I value all people for who and what they are

I tend not to be critical of others

I have succeeded in passing the Access course with distinction as a mature student

I put other people's needs before my own

I have two children and manage a home as a single parent, as well as caring for my father

I sing in a choir

Weaknesses

I tend to think that everyone is as enthusiastic as me

I am not very good at writing essays

I have never had success in formal examinations

I am not confident in my own abilities and tend to stay quiet

I am reserved with new people

I tend to retreat into the background in group situations

I am critical of myself and think I can't do things

Opportunities

I have a place on the course, support from my employer and my salary

I can use my previous experiences within the course and build on these

I can use the resources in college to build my academic skills, help me with my confidence building and assertiveness

I can use my placements to build up my skills in different areas

I have the maturity to acknowledge my limitations and ask for help and support

Barriers

Balancing and managing my time so that I can fit in everything that I need to do

Not having a computer at home and not having any IT skills

Looking after the children/dad

Travelling to college and placements

Choir practice

My lack of confidence in myself

My lack of assertiveness

The benefits in doing this at the start of a course is that we can actively and consciously use what we have discovered about ourselves in planning our strategies for the future. So the next step in this exercise is to form an action plan.

Part of the process of action planning is to be willing to think differently about something, and find ways of overcoming problems that you had not previously considered. In Jaz's case, for instance, she had always felt that her son's needs came first and that she needed to look after her father in the same ways that her mother had. As a result, she considered herself, and her needs as less important. She had got into the habit of doing all the housework because it was easier than nagging at the children or asking her father, and always spent Sunday evening doing the ironing in front of the television. However, she realized as a result of the SWOB analysis that there were ways in which she, the children, her dad and the situation would have to change if she was to be able to find the time to study at home.

She sat down with them all and together they worked out ways that they could each take some responsibility around the house, starting with a rota for the washing up and putting away after meals. All three took responsibility for keeping their rooms tidy. However, after thinking about it, Jaz realized that it was her problem that she wanted the rooms tidy, and not theirs! So, a compromise was negotiated so that the rooms they shared, especially the living room, would be kept tidy, and the boys could live in their rooms as they pleased, provided it did not interfere with anyone else. They also devised a rota for sharing out the washing, ironing and cleaning the bathroom, agreeing to rotate this every week. Jaz had to teach the boys to iron effectively, and they learned basic skills for feeding themselves and cooking simple meals for the whole family. Dad learnt how to manage the washing machine and to plan to sort the washing into types, do the loads and get them dry to prevent dirty or wet washing cluttering the house.

Previously, Jaz could not have conceived of expecting her boys or dad to take part in all the tasks that she felt were her responsibility as a mother. But, through the necessity of having to create more time in her busy life, she had to stand back and force herself to think about things in a different way. She realized that untidy bedrooms were not really that important – especially if she didn't go into them! She found very quickly that they would not go hungry if she did not have food on the table, and that in fact one of them was turning out to be a very good cook. She also realized that, while she needed to be more active as a housekeeper when the children were small, much of what she was doing she did out of habit, and she hadn't kept up with the boys' growth and abilities. Dad was turning out to be useful, and indeed taking pride in the tasks he was doing. In providing the boys with the opportunities to take more responsibility in the house she was facilitating them into adulthood and preparing them for a time when they too would live independently or with their own partners.

Jaz had turned what could have been a huge barrier to success into positive opportunities for herself and her family. Not only that, she found she had six hours per week extra study time – time that had previously simply disappeared into routine house work, which was still getting done but in a different way.

The necessity to find a solution to a problem, and using a potential barrier as a stimulus for changing her way of thinking, was also a positive learning experience for Jaz. It made her realize how she had got into the habit of thinking the ways she did and thought about things, were the only ways. A willingness to put aside the things we take for granted, or to reconsider things that we think are fixed and beyond our control, are the first steps in enabling our own personal development. They will also help us move in different ways of experiencing our lives.

Reflective activity

Work through all of the features that you identified in your SWOB analysis and formulate a plan of action from them.

First of all, plan to reinforce your strengths by making the most of your opportunities.

Next, think about your weaknesses. Many of these you may think are outside your control. But, when you consider it, they are your weaknesses, not anyone else's, and therefore it is only you that can do anything about them! Recognizing and taking responsibility for doing something about the things you don't like about yourself is a major step. Going a bit further and actually doing something about it is just one more! So, if you find yourself glossing over some of these, stop, consider why you are trying to avoid dealing with them and perhaps set yourself a challenge by tackling at least one.

Similarly, it is important to start making plans to tackle or overcome the barriers that you identified. As Jaz did, try to look at a problem in a different way to your normal perspective. If necessary, bounce the problem off another person to see whether they see it in a different way to you, or can propose a solution that you hadn't thought about.

The final step, of course, is to put the plan into action! And only you can decide to do that…

In completing this activity, you have taken the first steps in reflective practice. You have certainly completed the ERA reflective cycle, possibly several times if you have actually sorted out many of the issues that you had identified.

This illustrates that reflective practice is not simply confined to our professional practice. Using the techniques and strategies of reflective practice enables us to become more aware of the ways in which we live our lives and more open to the possibilities of alternatives and change.

Using reflection to identify our needs, and courses of action for the future, makes it a very positive strategy. This section also illustrates that reflection need not simply focus on a single incident, nor remain in the realms of the past – using reflection to inform the future is its most significant and valuable feature.

KEY POINTS

- Identifying our strengths helps us to value ourselves and build on these for the future
- Identifying our weaknesses allows us to plan to remedy them
- Identifying our opportunities ensures that we are aware of options available to us
- Identifying the barriers in our lives helps us to take a fresh look at where we are and how to change

Coping with challenges

Within your SWOB analysis it is likely that you drew attention to the ways in which you cope with challenges in your life. You may have identified these as both strengths and weaknesses. Look back on these now and consider whether you want to add more features in here.

Basically, just about anything that we do is a challenge, and we adopt very similar ways of tackling these, no matter what they are. On the whole, we manage these well, and as a result tend not to think of them as challenges at all – for instance, synchronizing a new phone with your computer or arranging to meet up with friends you haven't seen for a long time. The very fact that you have started your course means that you are successful in meeting the challenges of gaining the appropriate entry criteria, completing the application process successfully, surviving the selection process and turning up on the first day! Once we have done something successfully we tend to take it for granted and it becomes part of our past history. But, subconsciously, we are more likely to repeat behaviours that have been successful than those that haven't. We have these strategies as readily available resources, and just have to ensure we use these consciously when tackling challenges in the future.

In considering events and experiences to be challenges though, we often focus only on the negative things that happen to us, or the things that go wrong. These occur because the usual ways we cope with things have failed us. They tend to stay in our mind for longer and as a result we may start to believe we are not good at certain things or can't cope in certain situations. When confronted with a similar experience, we remember the ways we felt before and have a tendency to think the same will happen again.

Case study

Jaz's exam phobia

As one of her 'weaknesses' Jaz identified her inability in the past to pass exams. But, the fact that she had gained entry to the University programme gave her confidence that she had the academic ability to pass the course if she could overcome her previous experiences with exams. She decided to use this as the basis for her first reflective activity in her programme. She used the simple 5WH cues to guide the questions she asked herself.

What is the problem?

I've always performed badly in examinations. I never had time to do enough revision, didn't know what to revise and ended up doing very little. I was always so envious of those people who said they'd done no work but then managed to pass with good grades. I panic when I turn over the paper and see the questions and go blank. I start with the first question, then find I run out of time and end up rushing the rest of the questions and don't finish the paper. Sometimes I don't even answer all the questions or realize half way through that I've misunderstood what the question was asking and have to start again. I am terrified now of taking examinations and get into a state waiting for the exam room to open.

What do I want to achieve?

I know that exams are part of the assessment strategy through the four years of the programme and therefore I need to overcome my fear, take control and learn to cope with them as another challenge in life. I want to:

- Plan to pass the exam
- Conquer my exam nerves
- Utilize my coping skills and strategies to tackle this as a problem that is within my control.

What am I going to do?

- Ensure that I plan a revision timetable and stick to it
- Find out what is required in the exam
- Learn relaxation techniques and stress relief strategies that I can use to control anxiety and panic.

Who can I enlist to help me?

- My academic advisor, who will help me understand what is needed in the examination, what the structure is and what I need to do
- My sons and father, who need to help more in the house to enable me to have more time for revision
- My friends Sharee and Olugbenga who are on the course – we can set up a revision group and help support each other
- My study group on the programme as we can plan different ways to learn together other than trying to rote learn things which we then forget!.
- The choir will need to do without me for two weeks

- My practice mentor when examinations are related to practice work, such as patient/client care, drugs, etc.

When am I going to do this?

- I'll make an appointment with my academic advisor tomorrow
- I'll draw up a revision timetable over the weekend, and plan sessions with Sharee and Olugbenga to make the most of the time we have available
- Tomorrow, I'll find some old exam papers and ensure that I really know what is required so that I don't have any surprises in the exam room
- I'll have a word with Dad and the boys tonight
- I'll ring James, the choir leader, and explain my absence to him tonight.

Where am I going to do these things?

- I need to ensure I have quiet space and time at home
- I'm going to spend more time in the study areas at University, and avoid joining others for coffee in free periods, but study instead
- Sharee, Olugbenga and I can alternate studying in each other's homes so we can share their childcare and watching my dad
- I will go and see my academic advisor at the University.

How am I going to do achieve these?

- I realize now that the obstacles to passing exams are in my own head, and therefore the solutions are also within my control.
- I realize that I need to plan to **pass** examinations rather than leaving everything to chance – my mind set has to change, and consider exams as challenges rather than obstacles
- I need to make a plan and stick to it – it's under my control.

Jaz realized that when she looked at her previous exam experiences in a different way she was able to deal with them in the same way as she would when things (usually) worked out the way she wanted them to. By understanding the ways in which she would normally approach a situation, and being aware of this, she could plan to use them in a situation she found difficult.

Try the following activity yourself.

Reflective activity

1. Think back to the last time you organized a holiday.

   What did you do? Write a list of the stages and activities you went through in order to ensure your holiday happened as you wanted it to.

   Your approach to planning a holiday is probably typical of the ways in which you tackle most challenges you are able to predict. All of us will go about this in different ways but, on the whole, the strategies we adopt enable us to succeed. In recognizing these, and actively using them throughout your course, you are more likely to be successful.

2. Now, think about a challenge that took you by surprise – perhaps the washing machine broke down mid-cycle or the car engine started billowing steam while you were driving it.

   What did you do? This time, add in your memories of how this unexpected challenge made you feel, as well as how you dealt with it.

   Once we get over the initial shock of an unexpected challenge, we tend to use the same coping strategies as when we have time to forward plan. By analyzing your responses to things that hit you out of the blue, you will see how you are likely to react to these sort of events in your clinical practice.

Health care practice is characterized by the unexpected, and therefore you need to recognize the ways in which you deal with this. Often, the unexpected is not entirely unexpected – for instance you may predict that an elderly man who has had a stroke will be in danger of falling when getting out of bed. So, much of dealing with the unexpected relies on developing your underlying knowledge base so that you can predict possible events in the future and work to prevent these happening. Even so, some things will always happen when you least expect them, despite all your planning and precautions. You need to actively develop strategies that will enable you to function effectively in these situations. Clearly, your course and your supervisors in practice will help you. But there are many things you can do for yourself through planning to recognize and deal with your own reactions. By drawing on the ways that you know you have dealt with challenges successfully in the past, you will begin to eradicate behaviours that have prevented you from coping. For instance, panic reactions, such as running away and asking someone else to deal with things, are not going to develop your own confidence and competence as a practitioner!

Over to you

Actively recognizing the ways you cope with challenges, and planning to change any behaviour that prevents you from dealing with those challenges effectively is within your control.

1 Next time something happens that you see as a challenge, take note of how you feel, think and react.

2 Later, ask yourself what you did that was effective, and what was less so.

3 Think about these reactions and try to use more of those that are effective and change the negative responses in the future.

Having focused on yourself as a person, it is time to consider you as a practitioner.

KNOWING OURSELVES AS PRACTITIONERS

When we enter a profession we bring with us our own beliefs, values and perceptions of it we have developed over the years. For some reason, we have chosen to enter this particular profession, and often we have only a vague understanding of why this is.

However, the type of practitioner we become is dependent on these underpinning beliefs and values, and it is therefore worth taking some time to become aware of what they are.

Reflective activity

Choosing a professional specialty

What was it that attracted you to the health care specialty that you have entered? Try to think about this in terms of:

● the type of service you provide

● the knowledge and skills you will develop

● the type of work you will be doing

● the types of patient you will be dealing with

● the relationships you will have with your patients

● the amount of professional autonomy and independence you will have

● the environments in which you will work

● the relationships you will have with other professional groups

● your career prospects

● your previous experiences of the profession.

The answers that you have given in this activity will have painted a picture of your chosen professional group. This may have changed as a result of your experiences so far on your course, as you enter the real world of the profession as opposed to the one you imagined before. It will continue to change as you move through your educational preparation and as you gain the 'hands-on' experience that turns you from an onlooker to a practitioner in your own right. Your views are also likely to change once you have qualified and start to try out and use your knowledge and skills in a professional capacity. You will also be taking on the responsibilities of providing a safe and competent service for your patients, as well as being accountable for your own actions.

Where do our beliefs and values come from?

As soon as we start to become social beings we begin to learn the beliefs and values of our society. The socialization processes that we go through, from our early experiences at home, through our school years, college and into adulthood, all provide us with ideas about what is right and wrong, and what are acceptable attitudes and behaviour. There are many influences on us as we grow and mature into adulthood, and hence we absorb, unconsciously, the ways in which we view the world. As a result, when we enter professional education, we bring with us a pre-formed picture of the way the profession is. We also have a picture of the person who is a professional. These influences may come from:

- previous personal experience of the profession
- knowing someone in the profession
- media influences – TV, newspapers, films, books, magazines, advertising material
- careers information.

The pictures we have of our profession tend to be idealized and are not really a representation of the 'real-life' experience of the profession as it happens every day. Your views of the profession will be modified by the 'insider' experiences, as opposed to those of an outsider looking in. The influences that will help you develop your beliefs and values and gain a more realistic picture may come from:

- your own fundamental beliefs and values, derived from the culture you have grown up in
- your own personality, attitudes and approach to life
- other professionals – practitioners, educators
- codes of professional conduct
- societal ethical and moral codes and values.

Much of the way in which you learn these, and take on the attributes of your profession, will be through role modelling other practitioners. Identifying role models and thinking about what it is that makes them the type of

Accountable
Being able to justify our actions to others and take responsibility for them

Socialization processes
The interactions that we have with others that enable us to learn how to fit into different social situations, e.g. learning the rules of working in a specific profession

professional practitioner you admire, is a useful way of learning how to develop the characteristics of your professional group. All the practitioners you meet during your course will have some sort of impact on you. You will, probably quite unconsciously, select some of these as role models because you admire and respect the ways in which they conduct themselves as practitioners. On the other hand, you will identify some people as poor role models for you because their behaviour makes you feel uncomfortable in some way.

Reflective activity

What is a professional practitioner?

You can do this exercise either by yourself or with other people. Sometimes it is useful to work with others in this way, because they may see other things that you have not thought about and therefore you see a broader picture than one that you would have developed by yourself.

First of all, think about and list the characteristics of the type of person that you thought would be typical of a practitioner in your profession before you started your course. For instance, you might think about the way they look, or the way that they interact with other people. Have you a role model who, for instance, made you think about joining your profession? Or maybe you have seen portrayals on television of different kinds of health professional that gave you some ideas about how you think they work.

Now take some time to think about the attributes of a practitioner that you have already met and worked with that you admire. For instance:

- Initially, what was it that made them stand out for you?
- What is it about them that you want to be like?
- How do they interact and relate with patients?
- How do they interact and relate with other members of staff?
- How do they conduct themselves as a professional person? For instance, think about how they embody their code of professional conduct, how they maintain the confidentiality, respect and dignity for their patients
- How do they present themselves in terms of their speech, dress and ways of working?
- How knowledgeable are they about their practice?

Now think about someone who you do not admire, who perhaps has done something that stands out in your mind and makes you think that you do not want to be like them. Discuss their characteristics with a colleague, or note them down.

- What was it that they did that made you remember them?
- Why did you decide that you did not want to be like that?
- What standards can you use to assess their behaviour (e.g. the code of professional conduct, other professional standards, everyday expectations of the ways in which people deserve to be treated)

By now you will be building up a picture of the type of practitioner you want to become and also forming some ideas of the type that you don't want to be like. Engaging in reflective practice, using your clinical experiences, will help you recognize your own developing professional persona, and you will be able to constantly check that you are comfortable with the image you see emerging.

Throughout your course you will be challenged constantly by encountering practice that makes you feel uncomfortable. This might be because you are unhappy with the way that a person behaves, or it might be that you witness episodes of care that do not reach a safe standard. These episodes, while disappointing, because they dispel our illusions about professional practice, can also serve a useful purpose in helping us to recognize, and reinforce, our own underpinning professional values and beliefs.

By sharing your reflections on your experiences in health care you will be developing an understanding of your own values, beliefs and ideas about your chosen profession. You will also come to understand how other people can operate with a different set of ideas that, although not the same as yours, provides them with an effective starting point for their own practice. Despite the effects of education and experience in practice, we all develop our own unique set of beliefs and values that inform the ways in which we practise.

Most of these, for most people, fall within parameters that are considered acceptable. One of the purposes of allocating you to workplace supervisors is to help you to develop these acceptable beliefs and values, which will designate you as a person worthy of practising independently.

However, if people display unacceptable behaviour, either attitudinally or through their treatment of other people, they will be sanctioned.

As a student this may mean that your supervisors and lecturers help you to develop more appropriate ways of conducting yourself, or help you to see things in the way that is acceptable to your profession. In order to be accepted on to the professional register in some professions, your lecturers have to sign a declaration of 'good character'. All health care professional students have mentors or supervisors who assess practice skills and development, in addition to the assessments made by academic tutors. Nursing and midwifery students will also have 'sign-off mentor' who assesses performance during the final placement – similar judgements will be made for other health care professions as experienced practitioners are asked to assess your competence to practise by yourself in an independent capacity.

Workplace experience is a core component of all programmes for health care practitioner preparation, and ranges in length from a few weeks each year, to almost half the time. Thus, demonstrating that you have developed the attributes of your chosen professional group is vital in completing your course. Professional attitudes include not just your approach to the technical skills and knowledge of your profession, but also the way you accept the diversity of patients and clients you may come into contact with, valuing others and recognizing any prejudices you have and planning to overcome these when acting in a professional capacity. Without this acceptance of the professional values expected within your profession, and even if you have successfully passed all of your course components, you will be unable to register as a practitioner. This may happen, for instance, if you commit an illegal act, such as stealing from patients, display preferential treatment or exhibit prejudicial attitudes on the basis of race, gender, age, or sexual orientation, but can also occur if others do not approve of the way in which you act and can present a case against you. Once you have qualified and are on a professional register, you can be removed from that register if it is proved that you have contravened the code of professional conduct (NMC 2008, HPC 2004). This, of course, is the most serious penalty that can be imposed on you. However, your employer can dismiss you from your job for misconduct as well, and all employers have disciplinary processes that can be used to draw your attention to unacceptable behaviour.

In this section you will have developed a deeper understanding of your own beliefs about your profession and the people who work in it, and your own beliefs and values that underpin your role as a practitioner in your field. It is worth revisiting these at different stages in your course and comparing what you think then with what your initial impressions were. It will be interesting to see whether your views and perceptions change as you progress through your course. Ask yourself why this might be and whether you need to take stock of where you are at the time, re-thinking the ways in which you approach your practice.

Reflective activity

Myself as a practitioner

This is a challenging exercise as it asks you to really think about your own beliefs and values, which are contributing to the type of practitioner you will become. Try to complete the sentences below. This is a useful exercise to do with other people, and the trick here is to not look down the list of questions but to take them one by one.

1 As a student in the clinical environment, I like to be called......... because.........

2 My practice experience so far includes.........

3 I want to be a......... practitioner because.........

4 I believe I will be a good practitioner because.........

5 My philosophy of practice is.........

6 I believe that the most important part of my job is.........

7 I believe that good practitioners have the characteristics of.........

8 My relationship to my patient is as a.........

9 I carry out this relationship by.........

10 My status in regard to my patient is.........

11 The environment in which I am most effective in my job is.........

12 The environment in which I would like to do my job is.........

13 My definition of care is.........

14 The part I play in other people's care is.........

15 I achieve this by………

16 I understand holistic care to mean………

17 In my practice I achieve this by………

18 Some of my strengths as a practitioner are………

19 Some of my weaknesses are………

20 To become more effective as a practitioner I have to work on:

    a Understanding my philosophy of practice

    b Skills such as………

    c My theoretical approach

    d My personal growth

    e Other things such as………

21 The things that I need to learn in order for me to do this are………

22 I will achieve this by………

Now spend a few minutes reviewing what you have learnt from this exercise in terms of:

- Your own beliefs and values
- Other people's beliefs and values (if you have done this with others)
- How useful this has been as an exercise in helping you to identify your guiding principles
- Its usefulness as a reflective strategy
- What action you need to take as a result of the things you have learnt

KEY POINTS

- We all work as professionals from a distinct and individual values base.
- Many of these values come from our previous experiences of the profession.
- Many of these will come from our experiences of working with others.
- Recognizing our values is crucial to understanding who we are as practitioners and how we practise.

IDENTIFYING YOUR LEARNING STYLE

Just as we all have different personalities, so we all have preferences about the ways that we learn. Mostly these are unconscious: we don't usually deliberately choose the types of activity that suit us because we are, more often than not, unaware that some methods suit us and some don't. The purpose of this section is to help you to explore your past experiences of learning from a variety of situations in order to enable you to identify your learning style and recognize how this affects the way that you plan.

Most of the learning that we are aware of takes place in a formal learning situation where teaching and learning methods are not chosen by us but are imposed by others such as teachers, mentors and lecturers. Many of us find learning in these formal situations a challenge, and often one that we choose not to engage in once we leave school or college. Sometimes we may label ourselves as failures because we don't seem able to learn in the way others want us to, and we blame ourselves for not being able to cope with the material that is thrown at us.

However, being unable to learn in these situations is not necessarily a result of not being capable of doing the work, or learning the skill. It may be down to the teaching and learning approach that is used. It may simply be that you don't learn in that way! For instance, many people find it difficult to start with a theory and then apply it to practice. How many times have you said 'I don't know what you are talking about, just show me'. This often happens when you need to understand the theoretical basis for learning practical skills. For instance, some people are quite comfortable with learning the wiring diagram of a plug and then going and practising the skills. Others, however, want to be shown how to do it and then to go back to the theory afterwards. In formal learning situations, we tend to be faced with the theory of something first, and only once we have mastered this are we allowed to go and practise. If you find it difficult to learn in this way, if you are one of the people who need to 'see' something before they can understand, the formal methods of learning that are used may be preventing you from learning, or at least they may be contributing to any problems you may have.

In adult learning situations, such as university, evening classes or even college courses, it is likely that you will meet a variety of teaching and learning methods. They are designed to help everyone to select the methods that are most likely to help them to learn effectively in a way that suits them. The wide variety of learning and teaching methods now available, including e-learning, online delivery and the extensive use of simulation laboratories and practice environments and placements, mean that all students have the opportunity to develop their knowledge and skills in ways most appropriate to them. At university, it is likely that you will study in small groups as well as attend lectures and more traditional teaching methods. Small group work activities are likely to include reflective learning where you are asked to discuss experiences in practice and extend your understanding of them – these will not only develop your knowledge but also your reflective skills and capacity to learn independently from your experiences. This is vitally important in ensuring your placements are learning placements, not just work experience to gain a specific number of hours or cases.

Having an awareness of the ways in which we learn best, the ways that we would choose to learn if we were left to ourselves, helps us to select from these methods to maximize our opportunities.

Over to you

Think back over your learning experiences so far in your life. These will include both formal educational experiences, and also those less formal, where you have perhaps learned things at home, in your workplace, or in your leisure time.

Make a list of the types of activity that you have used, and find an example that you have used each for.

Now, for each one, write down what you liked about it and what you didn't, whether it involved some activity on your part or whether it was a largely passive technique.

Finally, think about how effective it was for you in helping you to learn, and whether you felt any emotional response when using it, such as excitement, frustration or anxiety. Give it a score out of ten for how comfortable you felt in using it overall.

In this exercise you have identified the types of situation that suit you best and those that you feel most comfortable with.

The basis of this is that we all have a 'preferred learning style'. What this means is that the basic underlying features of our personality make some ways of learning more suitable for us as an individual than others.

How to identify your learning style

The questionnaire below (Table 2.1) is designed to find out your preferred learning style(s). Over the years you have probably developed learning habits that help you benefit more from some experiences than from others. Since you are probably unaware of this, this questionnaire will help you to pinpoint your learning preferences so that you are in a better position to select learning experiences that suit your style. It was first designed by David Kolb in 1970 (Kolb, 1984). However, there are many models for assessing your learning style, and you may prefer a simpler one than Kolb's. The following website is a good start to find alternative methods **www.learning-styles-online.com**.

There is no time limit to this questionnaire, but it will probably take about 10–15 minutes. There are no right or wrong answers. Look at the four statements in each row and decide how they refer to you. Allocate four marks to the statement nearest to you, three to the second, two to the third and one to the statement least like you.

	a	b	c	d
			Table 2.1 The learning style inventory (Kolb, 1984)	
1	I like to get involved	I like to take my time before acting	I am particular about what I like	I like things to be useful
2	I like to try things out	I like to analyze things and break them down into parts	I am open to new experiences	I like to look at all sides of issues
3	I like to watch	I like to follow my feelings	I like to be doing things	I like to think about things
4	I accept people and situations the way they are	I like to be aware of what is around me	I like to evaluate	I like to take risks
5	I have gut feelings and hunches	I have a lot of questions	I am logical	I am hard working and get things done
6	I like concrete things I can see, feel, touch and smell	I like to be active	I like to observe	I like ideas and theories
7	I prefer learning in the here and now	I like to consider and reflect about them	I tend to think about the future	I like to see the results of my work
8	I have to try things out for myself	I rely on my own ideas	I rely on my own observations	I rely on my own feelings
9	I am quiet and reserved	I am energetic and enthusiastic	I tend to reason things out	I am responsible about things

Use the grid in Table 2.2 to summarize your score on the learning style inventory and fill in your total score for each column in the spaces below.

	Table 2.2 Scoring grid for learning styles inventory		
CE Concrete experience	**RO Reflective observation**	**AC Abstract conceptualization**	**AE Active experimentation**
1a	1b	2b	2a
2c	2d	3d	3c
3b	3a	4c	6b
4a	6c	6d	7d
8d	8c	8b	8a
9b	9a	9c	9d
Total	Total	Total	Total

Only put down the 'marks' asked for. You will notice that the marks for 1c and 1d are not asked. This is intended to stop 'patterning' and is not a mistake.

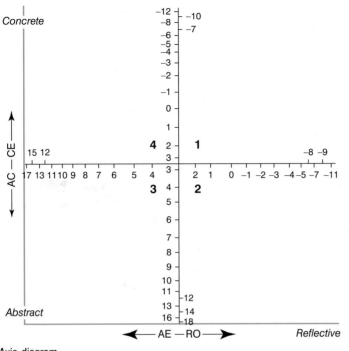

Figure 2.1   Axis diagram

Now use the scores you have from the four columns in the following way. First, subtract your RO score from your AE score.

Second, subtract your CE score from your AC score.

Plot the resulting figures on the two axes in Figure 2.1.

The four scores you originally arrived at can be plotted on to Figure 2.2 and joined up to produce your 'kite'.

The shape of your kite gives you a profile of your learning style and the ways in which you are likely to learn best. Kolb suggests that we collect and use our experiences in one of two ways:

- We can gather experiences first hand by 'living the experience' – Kolb calls this **concrete experience** (CE)
- We can gather experience second-hand by being told about or reading about it – Kolb calls this **abstract conceptualization** (AC).

The CE–AC axis is often called the Grasping Line.

We transform our experiences into knowledge again in one of two ways:

- We reflect on the experiences received in a considered and impartial manner. Kolb refers to this as **reflective observation** (RO)
- We are more concerned with seeking out the practical applications. Kolb calls this **active experimentation** (AE).

The RO–AE axis is often referred to as the Transforming Line.

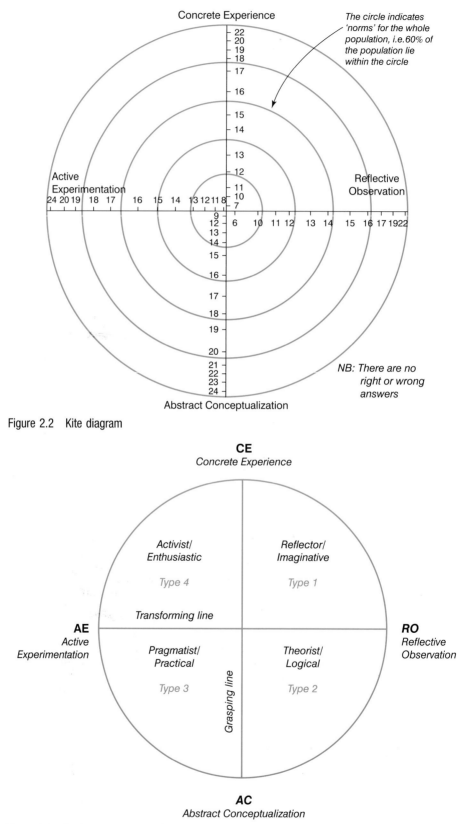

Figure 2.2   Kite diagram

Figure 2.3   Preferred learning styles quadrant

Preferred learning quadrant

The combination of scores on the kite indicates your preferred learning style. We all learn to grasp experiences and transform them into knowledge in all four ways. Combinations of preferred ways of grasping and transforming knowledge give rise to the preferred learning style which correspond to the quadrants in Figure 2.3 on the previous page.

No-one learns exclusively in just one style, but we all tend to fall mostly under the one descriptor and 'borrow' characteristics from the others. McCarthy (cited by Kolb, 1984) summarizes the four types of learner in Table 2.3.

Table 2.3 Types of learner (adapted from Kolb, 1984)	
Type four learner: Activist/Enthusiastic	**Type one learner: Reflector/Imaginative**
<ul><li>Integrates experience and application</li><li>Seeks hidden possibilities, excitement</li><li>Needs to know what can be done with things</li><li>Learns by trial and error, self-discovery</li><li>Seeks influence and solidarity</li><li>Enriches reality</li><li>Perceives information concretely and processes it actively</li><li>Is adaptable to change and relishes it, likes variety and excels in situations calling for flexibility</li><li>Tends to take risks, at ease with people, sometimes seen as pushy</li><li>Often reaches conclusions in the absence of logical justification</li><li>Functions by acting and testing experience</li></ul>**Strengths**: Action, carrying out plans **Goals**: To make things happen, to bring action to concepts **Favourite question**: What if?	<ul><li>Integrates experience with the 'self'</li><li>Seeks meaning, clarity and integrity</li><li>Needs to be personally involved</li><li>Seeks commitment</li><li>Learns by listening and sharing ideas</li><li>Values insight, thinking, works for harmony</li><li>Absorbs reality</li><li>Perceives information concretely and processes it reflectively</li><li>Interested in people and culture</li><li>Divergent thinkers who believe in their own experience and excel in viewing concrete situations from many perspectives</li><li>Model themselves on those they respect</li></ul>**Strengths**: Innovations and imagination. They are ideas people. They function through social integration and values clarification **Goals**: Self-involvement in important issues, bringing unity to diversity **Favourite question**: Why?
Type three learner: Pragmatist/Practical	**Type two learner: Theorist/Logical**
<ul><li>Practises and personalizes</li><li>Seeks usability, utility, solvency, results</li><li>Needs to know how things work</li><li>Learns by testing theories in ways that seem most sensible</li><li>Values strategic thinking, is skills-oriented</li><li>Edits reality</li><li>Perceives information abstractly and processes it actively</li><li>Uses factual data to build designed concepts, needs hands-on experiences, enjoys solving problems, resents being given answers</li><li>Restricts judgement to concrete things, has limited tolerance for 'fuzzy' ideas</li><li>Need to know how things they are asked to do will help in real life</li><li>Functions through inferences drawn from their bodies</li><li>They are decision makers</li></ul>**Strengths**: Practical application of ideas **Goals**: To bring their view of the present into line with future security **Favourite question**: How does this work?	<ul><li>Forms theories and concepts</li><li>Seeks facts and continuity</li><li>Needs to know what the experts think</li><li>Seeks goals attainment and personal effectiveness</li><li>Learns by thinking through ideas</li><li>Values sequential thinking, needs details</li><li>Forms reality</li><li>Perceives information and collects data</li><li>Thorough and industrious, re-examines facts if situations are perplexing</li><li>Enjoys traditional classrooms</li><li>Schools are designed for these learners</li><li>Functions by thinking things through and adapting to experts</li></ul>**Strengths**: Creating concepts and models **Goals**: Self-satisfaction and intellectual recognition **Favourite question**: What?

Recognizing our preferred learning style enables us to use it to learn more effectively. At the very least it helps us to understand why each person seems to learn better from different teaching and learning methods and why tutors should try to incorporate a range of methods into a course. While we all learn to adapt to the methods we need to use, some will find that they prefer one over another. Hence the reason that some people naturally seem to take to reflective processes and practices as learning strategies. Whereas others struggle to grasp even the fundamentals and find it more challenging.

Often we have no choice in the ways in which we learn: for instance, lectures, seminars and group work, and individual tutorials are always likely to be a feature of formal educational settings. However, there are times, particularly when you are working independently in clinical placements or have private study time, that you can choose the learning methods you use. This is where the predominance of your preferred style of learning is likely to come to the fore, and you will select methods that you feel most comfortable with, or even enjoy! Table 2.4 identifies the types of learning activity that people with each learning style are likely to gain the most from – and conversely, the type of activity least likely to engage them.

Which type of learner are YOU?

Table 2.4 Learning activities and learning styles				
	Type 4: Activist/ Enthusiastic	**Type 1: Reflector/ Imaginative**	**Type 3: Pragmatist/ Practical**	**Type 2: Theorist/ Logical**
Learns best from activities where:	There are new experiences, problems or opportunities Short 'here and now' activities are used, e.g. role play There is excitement, drama or crisis and a range of diverse activities to tackle They have the limelight, e.g. chairing meetings, leading discussions There is opportunity to generate ideas without the constraint of policy, structure or feasibility They are thrown in at the deep end with a task they think is difficult They are involved with other people It is appropriate to have a go	They are encouraged to watch, think and chew over activities They can stand back from events and listen and observe They can think before acting They can thoroughly research the problem They have the opportunity to review what has been learned They are asked to produce carefully considered analyses and reports They are helped to exchange ideas with other people without danger They can reach a decision in their own time without tight deadlines	There is an obvious link between the theory and the problem on the job They are shown techniques with obvious practical advantages They can try out and practise techniques with feedback from a credible expert They are exposed to a model they can emulate They are given techniques currently applicable to their job They are given immediate opportunity to implement what is learned There is validity in the learning activity, i.e. real problems They can concentrate on practical issues	What is being offered is part of a system, model, concept or theory They can explore the associations between ideas They can question and probe the basic assumptions or logic They are intellectually stretched They are in structured situations with a clear purpose They can listen to ideas that emphasize rationality and are well argued They can analyze and generalize the reasons for success or failure They are offered interesting ideas even though they are not immediately relevant They are required to understand and participate in complex situations

(Continued)

Table 2.4	Learning activities and learning styles (*Continued*)			
	Type 4: **Activist/** **Enthusiastic**	**Type 1:** **Reflector/** **Imaginative**	**Type 3:** **Pragmatist/** **Practical**	**Type 2:** **Theorist/** **Logical**
Learns least from activities where:	Learning involves a passive role They need to stand back and not be involved They are required to deal with a lot of 'messy' data They are involved in solitary work Theoretical statements are used The same activity is repeated over and over again There are precise instructions to follow with little room for manoeuvre They are asked to do a thorough job and attend to detail	They are forced into the limelight They are forced into situations that require action without planning They are thrown into something without warning They are given insufficient data on which to base a conclusion They are given cut and dried instructions on how things should be done In the interest of expediency, they have to make short cuts	There is no context or apparent purpose Emotions and feelings are emphasized They are involved in unstructured activities where ambiguity and uncertainty are high They are asked to decide without a basis in policy, principle or concept Learning is superficial They doubt that the subject matter is methodologically sound They find the subject matter shallow or gimmicky They feel out of tune with the other participants	The learning is not related to an immediate need Organizers of the learning seem distant from reality There is no practice or guidelines on how to do the task They feel that people are going round in circles and not getting anywhere fast enough There are political, managerial or personal obstacles to implementation They cannot see sufficient reward from the learning activity

Over to you

You might like to spend some time now considering the implications for yourself of identifying your preferred learning style and how you can plan to use that in your learning.

KEY POINTS

- Recognizing our preferred learning style is a short cut way to making the most of our learning experiences
- We can plan to use learning strategies that tie in with our preferred learning style
- As reflective learning from experience is self-dependent, we have choice and control over what strategies we use

IDENTIFYING YOUR WRITING STYLE

During your course you are going to be doing a lot of writing. This will take many forms and have different purposes. Underpinning these is the basic approach you take to writing, arising from your learning style and personality. It is worth thinking more about this because in understanding how we write we can make choices about the ways we use writing as a learning strategy in itself.

First of all, though, it's worth exploring where our feelings about writing come from. As with most of our ideas, our perceptions, attitudes and feelings about writing arise from the experiences we have had. Let's face it, we write every day, and for most of us the physical and psychological acts of writing have become second nature. We may, for instance, unhesitatingly write an e-mail or text to a friend. But there are other kinds of writing that evoke emotional responses, such as writing business letters, constructing an essay or sitting an examination.

Reflective activity

Think back over the past ten years and on the left hand side of your page write a list of the different types of writing that you have done in this time, leaving a few lines between each one – remember, texting, blogging, Facebook and tweeting are all types of writing.

On the other side of the page, for each type of writing that you listed, answer the following questions:

1 What was the purpose of writing?

2 Who were you writing for?

3 Who set the rules for that type of writing?

4 What part of it did you control and what components were controlled by others?

Our awareness of the different writing styles, dictated by the 'rules' for that particular style, enables us to select the one most appropriate to why we are writing. Look back over your list. How many of these were under the control of others or written according to 'rules' or conventions that you have learned in the past? Your list may look like this:

- Writing essays
- Writing presentations
- Writing research reports
- Records of patient/client care and interaction
- Recording observations
- Writing a job application
- Constructing a CV
- Writing for my professional portfolio
- Writing for my journal
- Sending emails

- Letters – for work, cover letters for job application
- Facebook updates
- Tweets
- Sending Christmas and birthday cards.

Rules for different forms of writing

This list is not exhaustive, but many of these have certain 'rules' that define what is supposed to be acceptable in that type of written communication. While there is room for individual style within these, we learn the difference, for instance, between writing an e-mail to a friend and writing an e-mail to complain or for a job application. On the whole, these rules serve positive purposes in enabling us to operate within the various roles that we lead in our lives. By knowing what is expected and what is not, we can operate within a safety zone, where we present the public side of ourselves to others.

Some of the types of writing, such as updating your Facebook page, you might not have thought of as writing because we are so comfortable with them that we don't think of them as writing at all; they arouse no fear or apprehension in us and therefore become automatic. Yet they still serve very important purposes in our lives and enable us to remember things, to communicate with others or to organize our lives in a particular way. While the rules for these are not so apparent, we still work within certain conventions, many of which we set up for ourselves. For instance, when texting you probably use abbreviations that you wouldn't use in your other forms of writing.

So, why do some rules for writing appear so intimidating, while others are simply part of the way we are? Part of the explanation here has to do with familiarity – the more we do, the easier it becomes. Other examples of this in other areas of our lives are learning to drive a car or ride a bicycle. We get to the stage where we do things without consciously thinking about them: to a certain extent, automatic pilot takes over. At first, everything you do appears to be governed by rules that you have yet to take on board and internalize as part of the way you work. These rules need to be learned and, once they are, they make your life easier.

If you successfully learn the rules of essay writing, for instance, it is more likely that you will have success in what you achieve. In terms of reflective writing, there is tremendous scope for creating your own rules and strategies as well as using those already created by others.

What kind of writer are you?

We often think that the way that we do things is the way that everyone does them.

Understanding how and why we write enables us to select ways of writing that may help us in reflecting. Sharples (1999) suggests that writers can be divided by the two broad approaches that they take to their writing – Discoverers and Planners. The characteristics of each type are shown in Table 2.5.

Table 2.5 The characteristics of each personality type for writing	
Discoverers	**Planners**
Driven by engagement with the text. For them, self-understanding arises from writing. They may prefer to begin by scribbling out a draft that reveals their thoughts to them. Then, they often rework their text many times, reading and revising until it 'shapes up' to the constraints of the task and audience. The rhythm of their writing is often one of long periods of engaged composing, followed by extensive revision.	Driven by reflection. For these people, writing flows from understanding. They spend a large proportion of their time on exploring ideas and on preparing mental or written plans. The plans guide composing and when there is a mismatch they either edit the text or revise the plan. Their rhythm of composing is, typically, one of rapid alternation between engagement and reflection, continually making minor adjustments to keep plan and text in harmony.

It is, of course, rare that we would all fall neatly into one category or the other. But, you may recognize some of your own characteristics from these descriptions.

But how will this help with your writing? By recognizing the ways that we have approached writing in the past, we can anticipate the ways in which we can make writing work for us. Equally, we can weigh up different ways of approaching writing and make a reasoned decision that some of them are not for us. This is really important in being comfortable with your writing, in choosing to write rather than being compelled to write because you are expected to. By understanding your own relationship with writing you are more likely to view it as a positive way of learning rather than something that is imposed upon you by an outside force.

Sharples (1999) goes further in his identification of writing styles by citing a study by Wyllie (1993) who looked at student and academic writers and attempted to classify them by the strategies they used as writers. This is shown in Table 2.6.

Table 2.6 Classification of writing strategies (adapted from Sharples, 1999, from original work by Wyllie, 1993)					
Writing characteristics	**Water colourist**	**Architect**	**Bricklayer**	**Sketcher**	**Oil painter**
Overall type of writer	*Planner*	*Planner (external)*	*Planner/ discoverer*	*Discoverer/ planner*	*Discoverer*
Strategy for writing	Single draft of whole paper with minimal revision, usually sequential	Plan mostly before writing, then write, then review	Rough plan, revise later	Polish one sentence, paragraph or section before moving to the next	Jot down ideas as they occur, organize later, rarely sequential

(Continued)

Table 2.6   Classification of writing strategies (adapted from Sharples, 1999, from original work by Wyllie, 1993) (*Continued*)

Writing characteristics	Water colourist	Architect	Bricklayer	Sketcher	Oil painter
Strategy for planning	Plan in head with broad headings	Detailed plan, composes with broad headings	Type of planning depends on combination of strategies	Composes with broad headings	Composes with broad headings. Sometimes have a rough plan
Order of writing	Always sequential	Often sequential	Sometimes sequential	Sometimes sequential, sometimes jumps about	Sometimes sequential, sometimes jumps about
Starting writing	Rarely start easiest part first	Sometimes starts easiest part first	Rarely starts easiest part first	Occasionally starts the easiest part first	Often starts easiest part first
Revision strategy	Little revision – some changes	Revises a fair amount, mainly at sentence level	Fair amount of revision, mainly spelling, grammar and re-sequencing	Much revision, mainly meaning and sequence changes, and sentence level	Much revision, particularly meaning and sentence
Correction strategy	Tends not to correct	Rarely corrects as they go, mainly corrects on printout	Corrects at both stages, but mainly later	Corrects as they go, also later	Corrects as they go, but mainly later
Strategy for reviewing work	Tends to review more on screen than other strategies	Tends to review on printout	Will review on screen, but prefer printout	Reviews on screen and on printout	Least tendency to review on screen, mainly printout
Relationship with screen	Doesn't find screen restrictive; rarely loses overall sense of the text	Occasionally finds screen too restrictive	Often finds screen restrictive. Often loses overall sense of the text	Occasionally finds screen restrictive	Occasionally finds screen restrictive

Reflective activity

Think about the ways that you approach your writing. Using Tables 2.5 and 2.6, tick the features that most apply to you. By counting the ticks you'll identify your overall approach to writing and understand the tendencies you adopt most commonly.

Table 2.6 illustrates what we all really know at heart – that different people approach writing in different ways. But sometimes we need reminding of this. Why do some people appear to sit effortlessly at a word processor, or with pen and paper in front of them, and write thousands of words, when the rest of us make just one more cup of coffee or hang another load of washing on the line, putting off the moment when we have to sit down with an empty screen in front of us! The different strategies identified by Wyllie may help us to understand the creative processes we use in writing. In order to accept that we can all be equally successful in writing we need to find a way of writing that suits us, rather than attempting to conform to one that someone else imposes.

If you pick the wrong approach for you,
it's all too easy to delay writing.

Reflective activity

Return to the list of types of writing in the first activity. For each one, identify whether you enjoyed this type of writing, whether you disliked it or whether you have no real emotion about it.

Think about the types of writing you have enjoyed in the past. These might be where you have got pleasure or satisfaction from writing or where you have gained from the experience of writing, even although the actual act of doing it may have been difficult for you. What was it about these that made them enjoyable?

Now consider the list of the types of writing that you don't enjoy. What is it about these that you don't like?

Knowing the reasons why you have enjoyed writing are important because you can plan to write reflectively in a style that suits you, and you feel comfortable with. For instance, if you like to write with a definite structure to your writing that has been framed for you, you may like to utilize one or more of the reflective strategies outlined in this book. This brings us back to whether you fall into the category of being a discoverer or a planner. For many people the idea of writing to a pre-determined structure is what puts them off, because they find it difficult to reduce their experiences into categories. For them, the types of writing that depend on creating a self-made structure, such as writing a letter, a story or a poem, or using more visual forms of writing such as mind maps, might be more attractive. Similarly, you may find that one single strategy is not appropriate for all writing occasions, and it is useful to consider trying other ways of writing that appear to be better suited to what you are writing about. Figure 2.4 shows Lioba's mind map, created when she was planning an essay on supporting women in labour (Lioba is a 2nd year midwifery student).

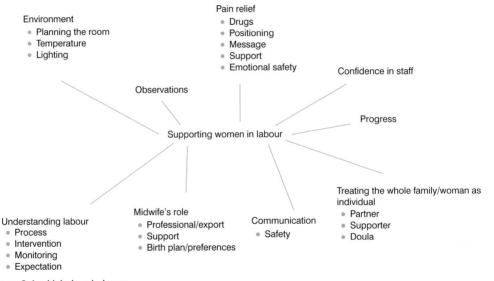

Figure 2.4   Lioba's mind map

Choosing to write reflectively

Writing can be used as a strategy in itself for reflection. In this case remember that it is the reflective component that is key here – that in writing reflectively you are writing to learn; to enable you to take another perspective. This is hard work; you will be deliberately deciding to explore your own reality and own experiences and at times this may be painful or reveal things to you that have previously been hidden. Equally, there can be great joy in writing, when we unlock secrets that have puzzled us for some time, or that we learn things about ourselves and those around us that we like and can celebrate. You will find strategies for reflective writing in Chapter 5.

Challenges to writing

We often have a reluctance to write – think back to that list of types of writing that you didn't enjoy and the reasons you gave for these. There are numerous reasons why we might put up barriers to writing, and unless you write habitually through choice, for instance keeping a diary, the act of writing tends to be something that we do because others tell us to do it. There are many barriers (and often excuses!) that we put up about writing, which we allow to inhibit us in seeing writing as a positive strategy for learning. Some of the reasons for this lie in the features of writing that we perceive to be outside of our control.

Rules for writing

We talked earlier about the 'rules' of writing. We may have been put off writing as a result of 'rules' being externally imposed – rules such as what you are expected to write about and how you are supposed to write it. This means that the writing tended not to be under our own control, we were writing to a formula that wasn't really very satisfying because it lacked an individual component.

Our experiences of writing are mainly a result of our past educational experiences or our need to write within the confines in our professional role – we learned to write for other people, and we write what others want us to write in the style others expect. In other words, we learn-to-write through the processes of socialization and teaching. These serve important purposes in enabling us to achieve what we need in order to get to the next stage in our lives, such as passing exams or successfully applying for a job, where we need to know the specific rules of writing in that particular setting. We learn the externally imposed rules of writing for other people but don't necessarily develop our own writing style.

You will also have been 'taught' the rules of writing as a formal process for communication – these rules become so ingrained that it is difficult for us to conceive of writing we can understand if it doesn't follow these rules. For instance, think back to the first time you opened a set of case notes. They would have been written in an order, and often language, that was not familiar to you, and thus you probably understood very little of what was written. However, once the conventions being used were explained to you, you would be able to make more sense of them, and eventually adopt the same sort of writing style yourself. So we are taught not only how to write but the ways in which to write it and often even what to write. This is because writing for this purpose becomes a medium of communication, so all people reading the notes and adding to them need to understand the set of rules governing the writing used in them.

Earlier, we asked you to identify as many types of writing as you could that were governed by different rules. Can you now add to these? The rules can be seen in a positive as well as a negative way because, once we understand them, they provide us with the structure and boundaries for what we write in a certain situation. These are useful, because they mean that anyone who knows the rules can understand what is expected and what is written. For instance, once you learn the rules of deciphering essay questions, and how essays are structured, then you will have little difficulty in writing work that gains a pass grade. At other times, however, you may be able to write without rules, such as when you are writing only for yourself and no-one else is likely to see the result. You may also have the freedom of writing where you define the structure, because you are not expected to conform to a given way of writing – this might be in a learning journal or a diary, for instance. Although others may read this, they do not have the power to ask you to write in a particular way.

In writing reflectively, as part of your reflective practice, you will meet all three approaches. In required course work, for instance, you may be asked to use a particular framework for reflection, or the choice may be left to you, with the proviso that you do use a recognized strategy. You may also be required to keep a learning journal, or portfolio, that is structured in a specific way and is used by all the people on your course. This is usually done so that you can concentrate on the reflective activity itself rather than having to find a structure to your writing as well. As you get to the later stages in the course, and you are more familiar with what you are doing in terms of having 'learned the rules' of the reflective process, you may be able to select alternative ways of writing reflectively.

However, you may also be writing reflectively in private. And here there are no rules other than the ones that you impose on yourself. Many students, especially when they are starting out, choose to use a specific strategy or framework. Others, however, may write instinctively as it suits them. This all comes back to the kind of writing style you have. The important criterion is that, no matter what you select in terms of your rules for writing, it should help you to achieve what you need to.

Writing for others – learning-to-write or writing-to-learn?

Allen *et al.* (1989) suggest that we *learn-to-write* primarily for other people, not for ourselves. This can be seen as fundamental to why many of us do not see the value of writing reflectively. Our previous experiences of writing have been rooted in providing some sort of evidence to others that we have learned something. This is opposite to the concept that writing might be useful in helping us to understand the world through a creative process of writing for ourselves in other word – writing-to-learn. The features of both of these paradigms are captured in Table 2.7.

Table 2.7 The two writing paradigms	
Learning to write	**Writing to learn**
• We can learn content whether or not we can write well • Writing and thinking involve different skills; therefore one is not necessarily linked to the other • Knowing something logically comes before writing about it • Writing is a sequential, linear activity that involves mastery of components such as sentence construction or outlining • Communication is the main purpose of writing; therefore, for students, written work is a product in which the student reports what he or she already knows • The student's audience is most often assumed to be the teacher.	• Writing is a process through which content is learned or understood (as opposed to memorized or reported) • Writing skills are primarily thinking skills (competence in one is inseparable from competence in the other) • Writing is a process of developing an understanding or coming to know something • Writing is a dialectical, recursive process rather than a linear or sequential one • Higher order conceptual skills can only evolve through a writing process in which the writer engages in an active, on-going dialogue with him or herself and others – learning and discovery are purposes as important for writing as communication • Different disciplines use different conceptual processes and thus have different standards for writing. Students can best learn writing within their own disciplines while writing for real, concrete audiences.

Adapted from Allen *et al.* 1989, p. 7

Learning to write The above paradigms explain a great deal in terms of understanding why writing is, for most of us, not an activity that we use creatively in our learning. Writing is usually an end point, when we finally pull all our reading and thinking together into an essay or other form of writing that will be given to others for their assessment and approval. None of the features in this list involves students writing for themselves other than to achieve an endpoint for which they will get credit; hence, to some extent, writing may be seen as something that is not for us at all and is only done when others demand it of us. In fact, it might not even be viewed as a useful activity, other than as a part of passing course components as a means to an end – a necessary evil to be got through and then not done again unless others require it.

For most of us, our experiences of writing are located within this *learning-to-write* paradigm. On the whole, we wrote what we thought others wanted us to write – for instance we would rewrite from textbooks or paraphrase from online sources in order to show a teacher that we had read (but not necessarily understood or learned) the material; or we would write an exam

Dialectical
The nature of logical argument

Recursive
Using a rule or procedure that can be applied repeatedly

Paradigm
A collection of features that together provide a particular view on something, e.g. the quantitative and qualitative paradigms in research

paper to prove that we could remember what we had read or been told. At times you may have written an essay with a title that asked you to discuss ideas, or analyze, or even be creative – but the title might have been given to you by someone else. Moreover, your success would have been dependent upon you correctly decoding the unseen rules about what was being asked of you – for instance, how many times have you been pleased with an essay, only to have it returned with a disappointing grade and the comment 'You haven't answered the question'. The *learning-to-write* paradigm assumes that thinking and writing are separate and different processes and that writing is simply a means to an end, not the end in itself.

Reflective activity

Why do you do what you do?

Think back to your school days. Try to describe your attitude to writing as a child. Why did you write, who did you write for?

What are the messages that your childhood experiences have given you about the value and purpose of writing that you have carried with you into your adult life?

Now think about your educational experiences, and other writing that you have done since school. Did this reinforce those previous experiences of writing, or enable you to develop different skills?

What is your attitude to writing now?

Writing to learn There is another way of looking at writing that enables us to see it as under our control and writing for ourselves. It is this attitude that enables us to use writing as a personal strategy for learning from our experiences, as opposed to the writing that we do for others.

The *writing-to-learn* view suggests that the very process of writing is a way of learning. This assumes that writing and thinking happen at the same time; that writing comes from thinking and that creativity arises from thinking about and doing writing. An important point here is that the *writing-to-learn* paradigm links understanding with writing. It suggests that we learn as a result of interacting with the subject matter and that in the process this material becomes transformed into 'knowing'. Thus, the very process of writing is not seen as a passive activity but is dynamic and leads to new connections being made and new understanding occurring.

These features are important when we see reflective writing as part of our strategy for learning about our practice in a professional capacity, because they acknowledge the individual nature of writing for each person. They remove the idea of writing from the basic idea of writing for others, producing a way of combining thinking and writing in a dialogue with ourselves to develop our understanding and create knowledge out of our experience.

We need, therefore, to see writing as being under our own control, and to see that we write for ourselves, not for other people. This is a major shift in perception for the majority of people and you will not necessarily be able to shrug off all your previous conditioning easily. You will still find yourself asking 'But what does the lecturer want me to write?' rather than 'What do I need to write to ensure that I understand?' Writing for ourselves is a big step forward, but writing as part of reflective practice does provide some freedoms and ways of helping you to shift from the *learning-to-write* paradigm to the *writing-to-learn* paradigm.

Case study

Cas

Cas is a second year, single midwifery student aged 24, entering her fourth semester of study on a three year degree programme.

Cas was fed up with getting marks that just passed – she wanted to improve her grades in academic work to match the higher assessments she was receiving in her midwifery practice. She knew that she put all the effort she could into writing her essays – she analyzed the titles deeply, did a lot of reading around the subject and tried to anticipate what the marker might be looking for. Yet, it was demoralizing to continually get feedback saying 'What do you think?', or 'What conclusions can you draw from this?' Surely, her view wasn't relevant, it was more important to show the marker that she knew the knowledge base? She discussed this with her tutor, who explained that part of becoming an independent practitioner was to be able to analyze what she was reading critically, and to demonstrate that she had weighed up the arguments and was able to make a judgement. She needed to show that she was able to draw together a range of perspectives and draw conclusions as a result, based on the evidence being presented. In so doing, she would demonstrate to her marker not only that she had read the material, but also that she understood it and could relate it to her own practice.

Cas decided to take a different approach to her next assignment. Instead of asking 'What does the marker want? she asked herself, 'What do I need to understand in order to practice more effectively?' This change of focus, from externally-driven to internally-motivated activity, enabled her to consider what she was reading in relation to midwifery practice, and translate that underpinning knowledge into something meaningful for her. In turn, she was able to relate her new knowledge to practice situations with women in labour, and found that she learnt through writing this up for the assignment. She also found that writing was easier, because she was dealing with what was real to her, rather than trying to write in what she thought was an 'academic' way. She was delighted to receive a higher mark for this work, and also with the comments which suggested she was now linking theoretical knowledge to the realities of midwifery practice.

Over to you

To unlearn things that have become part of us is very difficult and needs positive action on the part of the person involved. First of all, you need to have a desire to change, a willingness to do so and the motivation, or need, to carry it out. Seeing writing as something that you do for yourself is very difficult if all you have ever done is write for other people.

If you want to change, however, and see writing as a tool for learning, you can do so. It takes hard mental activity to change the way you approach a writing task. But conscious activity can do this, if you not only want to change but take the active steps to do so. Start by carrying a small notebook around with you and noting down things that puzzle or challenge you; or alternatively, each day, choose a different focus so that you don't get into the habit of doing the same thing all the time. Then, at the end of the day, or the first quiet time you get the next day, review your notes and write down alternatives or options to the problems. Use your writing purposively to explore your experiences and help you value, or sort out, things that have happened to you. Record the way you feel about things, and explore why you might have felt this way. Make writing your friend – it is there to help you, and is always on your side; writing seen in this way, can help you prevent mistakes, and act as a sounding board for taking action, trying out ideas, and sorting out problems before you take public action.

Getting it right

Resulting from the rules we learn, and writing for others, we absorb ideas about writing being right or wrong that influence us throughout our lives. These ideas are amazingly persistent and act as a barrier when we start writing reflectively. If your writing has only ever been for others to read, and this has been judged in some way, it is difficult to conceive of it in a different way. To see writing as value-free, as neither right nor wrong – it is by you, for you, and no-one else's judgement matters – is a tremendous change to the ways most of us have been used to writing. One of the most challenging tasks for educators is helping people to overcome the anxiety that makes them ask 'Am I doing it right?' or 'Is this what you want?' and enabling them to set their own parameters, outcomes and objectives in order to plan to achieve what they need.

As a student starting out in reflective practice, your writing will be a key indicator to those who are guiding and helping you in assessing whether you are achieving your goals. It is also key to you being able to assess your progress! One of the reasons that you may be constrained in your reflective writing initially will be because others need to be able to see that you have understood the principles of reflective writing and can use them to make sense of your experiences in practice. Learning to use the ERA reflective cycle is crucial to your development towards accountable and competent professional practice. So, although there may initially be a need to 'get it right', as you progress and are able to use the processes themselves you will find that this ceases to be a problem. In fact, you will start to define 'right' in your own terms, as opposed to those of other people, as you decide to take action as a result of your reflective activities. Hence, what is perceived as right is not necessarily appropriate at all, and the idea becomes redundant. What matters from our written reflective activity is that we learn from doing it – and therefore the activity will always be right!

What is likely to be an on-going hurdle, though, is turning your reflections into action.

Failure to complete the reflective cycle

This often occurs because when we start writing reflectively we are in the early stages of our academic careers and are only expected to write descriptively. While stopping at this stage is acceptable if you are practising using the reflective processes, in order for this to move to reflective practice you need to move to the final ERA stage of taking action.

You may see writing as an endpoint in itself and, if it does not achieve anything, you might consider it to be a waste of time. For instance, although writing essays may appear boring and repetitious, at least you are gaining academic credit for them and they contribute to your course completion. It is more difficult to see the purpose of writing learning journals or reflective reviews if these are not used in any constructive way.

Making the private public

The main thing to remember here is that you do not have to show your writing to anyone else. So you have choices to make when selecting the topics that you reflect about. These decisions depend on:

- Who is going to see the writing
- The purpose of the writing
- Whether the incident involves just yourself or other people
- Whether the writing includes private emotions or feelings.

Writing for an assignment that will be seen by other people is considered to be public writing. You therefore need to consider what you are going to write about, what the content of this is and whether you really want other people to know what your thoughts and feelings were. The people reading it will probably be making judgements about you that you do not want to share with others on the basis of this work – do you really want to provide information that might show you in a negative light? Despite the fact that critical incidents are chosen for their learning potential, there is a crucial difference between an incident in which you felt uncomfortable or inadequate, and one in which your behaviour and actions could be regarded as negligence or professional misconduct. So, it is prudent to think very carefully about the subject matter and content of any writing that is going to be made public before you embark on it.

The place for material of this sort is in your own reflective writing that you do for your own learning. This issue is very closely linked with the next one.

Writing things down that might have further consequences

Many critical incidents involve actions and behaviour that could be seen as unprofessional or, worse, resulted in damage or poor care for patients. Remember that all qualified staff are bound by a code of professional conduct and that they are duty-bound to take action should incidents come to their attention that break that code. This can happen unwittingly when students decide to describe incidents that they have witnessed that involved negligence or misconduct.

We deal with these two issues in more detail in Chapter 6.

The combination of the public nature of writing and the fact that there may be consequences arising from this mean that the selection of topics for reflective writing activities needs careful thought beforehand.

Reflective activity

Think about all of the things that have happened to you in your practice placement recently. Divide these into four groups headed:

- Experiences that I would be happy to use for an assignment
- Experiences that I would be happy to share only with my supervisor or academic staff
- Experiences that I would share with student colleagues or friends/family
- Experiences that I would keep private

Give reasons for your groupings.

Getting started

Writer's block happens to just about everyone, and unfortunately there are no easy ways of overcoming it. It may seem trite but, at the end of the day, the only thing to do is to start writing!

Perhaps one way of approaching this cognitively is to return to Wyllie's features of different types of writer. It is clearly no use in advising 'water-colourists' to write a detailed essay plan, as they tend to plan in their heads. Instead, an approach might be to talk through with another person the ideas that they have and the broad headings that could be used to structure their writing. As they have a tendency to write sequentially once they have the plan in their heads, they will probably be able to sit down and write straight away. In contrast, an 'architect' will have to have a very detailed plan before s/he starts to write in a structured way. The trick is to move from the planning stage to the writing stage, and various strategies can be used to do this.

For people who have detailed written plans, one strategy may be to simply write more and more detailed plans! In this way the brain is tricked into thinking it is still planning and the fear of writing therefore isn't experienced until a large part of the writing is done and it is too late. Another strategy is to write one section at a time, which can appear less daunting. If, for instance, you see a 3000 word essay as a series of sections each of about 500 words, it seems a much smaller task. This can be added to by creating subheadings, so that you can see how far you have got. It also provides a way of giving yourself rewards, as you may say 'I'll stop when I have finished that section' or 'I'll make a cup of coffee when I've got to the end of that topic'.

Alternatively, if you are a visual person, creating a one-page mind map for your writing may be a useful starting point. The mind map below shows the ways in which Cas, in the case study above, planned her assignment.. It many ways, it represents a detailed plan of an assignment, but contains all the key concepts and shows where links might be made. Each element forms a part of the whole, and therefore building up each main concept in sequential mind maps makes the work grow and leads, eventually, to writing.

Another way to start writing is to set a timetable. This approach is for the very pragmatic, practical sort of person who is able to clear their head and simply sit and write to a time schedule. Professional writers often do this – writing for instance to a fixed pattern between 6am and 10am. For those of us with hectic lives and many calls on our time, writing needs to be fitted in wherever there are a few hours of peace and quiet. This might be early in the morning before others get up, or late at night after the children have gone to bed. But reserving the space to write and knowing that you have to do it, are good motivators.

Finally, creating the mental space and incentive is important. Again, different personality types will achieve this by using differing strategies. Some people can simply ignore all the other things they need to do because they have prioritized their writing, and disregard the consequences. For others, prioritization incorporates other components of their life, and they find they cannot clear a mental space until the other commitments have been fulfilled. You will know what suits you best by reflecting on the ways that you usually start your writing.

However, other than passing on anecdotes, it is difficult to offer advice about writer's block. Sometimes, it is solved simply by the adrenaline released when you realize that the deadline for submission is looming and you simply have no choice but to sit down and do it!

Finding something to write about

Finding an issue that we can use to write about is often a barrier to getting started. It is also used as prevarication too! You will have been given an assignment brief if your work is to be assessed, and this will give you some clues as to the sort of topic that you can choose. Others will come from the criteria that you need to think about in selecting something suitable for reflection and the purpose for which you are reflecting. At other times, a critical incident will stand out in some way and stick in your mind until you do something about it.

Reflective activity

Return to the list you made in the previous activity. Think about each one of these and decide whether you would select it to reflect on if you were searching for a topic.

- What have you based your decisions on?
- For those that you have selected, what made them stand out for you?
- What kind of written reflection would you use them for: public or private?
- Would you use these as a focus for an assignment, a reflective review or critical incident analysis, or as part of a learning journal or diary?
- Why?

Once we see these barriers as challenges, it becomes easier to overcome them. The use of reflective thinking, and working out alternatives to the ways we usually see and do things, is the first step in this process. To use writing reflectively within our learning and professional practice we need to see it as a positive strategy for our development.

Reflective activity

Take some time now to consider the ways in which you approach writing. Think about each of the challenges that we have identified in the last section and ask yourself:

- What is my belief about this?
- Do I want/need to change this in order to be effective as a reflective writer?
- What changes could I make?
- What changes will I make?

KEY POINTS

- Our attitudes to writing are formed as a result of our previous experiences

- These are pervasive and tend to influence how we use writing within our learning

- Learning to approach writing through the principles of the writing-to-learn paradigm can facilitate us in using writing as a learning strategy

- There are no right and wrong ways of writing when we write for ourselves

- Identifying and understanding our writing style enables us to use it creatively

- There are many challenges to writing that get in the way if we let them

- Taking a proactive approach to writing helps us to overcome these

Proactive
Seeking things out

CONCLUSIONS

In working through this chapter we hope that you have come to know a little more about yourself than when you first opened this book.

You will have started thinking about the ways in which you approach life and learning, and about your attitudes and beliefs about your chosen profession. Hopefully, you will have begun to plan ways in which you can use all of these to maximize your learning opportunities throughout your course.

However, what you have also started to do is begin your career as a reflective practitioner. While you have not yet been asked to reflect on your experiences through a formal reflective framework of any sort, you have started to see how cue questions that ask you to focus on particular aspects of your experiences can be used to help you learn from them and make plans for the future. So...

Welcome to Reflective Practice!

RAPID RECAP

Check your progress so far by working through each of the following questions.

1 What is a SWOB analysis?

2 Where do our professional values come from?

3 How can knowing your preferred learning style help you to learn more effectively?

4 What are the challenges to using writing to learn?

If you have difficulty with more than one of the questions, read through the section again to refresh your understanding before moving on.

REFERENCES

Allen, D.G., Bowers, B. and Diekelmann, N. (1989) Writing to learn: a reconceptualisation of thinking and writing in the nursing curriculum. *Journal of Nursing Education*, **28**, 6–11.

Health Professions Council (2004) *Standards of Conduct, Performance and Ethics*. HPC, London.

Kolb, D.A. (1984) *Experiential Learning: Experience as the source of learning and development*. Prentice Hall, Englewood Cliffs, NJ.

Nursing and Midwifery Council (2008) *The NMC Code of Professional Conduct: Standards for Conduct, Performance and Ethics for Nurses and Midwives*. NMC, London.

Sharples, M. (1999) *How We Write*. Routledge, London.

Wyllie, R. (1993) *On the road to discovery: a study of the composing strategies of academic writers using the word processor*. University of Lancaster, MA thesis. www.learning-styles-online.com

CHAPTER 3
FRAMEWORKS FOR REFLECTION

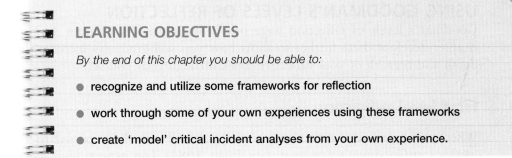

LEARNING OBJECTIVES

By the end of this chapter you should be able to:

● recognize and utilize some frameworks for reflection

● work through some of your own experiences using these frameworks

● create 'model' critical incident analyses from your own experience.

I n this chapter structures and strategies for reflection that you can use with other people or by yourself are introduced. These are all called 'frameworks' to avoid confusion. Although this is quite a theoretical chapter, each framework will be illustrated with examples to enable you to see how it works in practice. I will also be analyzing the frameworks that I use, so you can see how they have arisen, the ways in which they can be used and how they compare to each other. You'll see that structures and strategies can be useful as a guide, especially when starting out, because they provide cues, and ways of breaking experiences down that may be new to you. But all of these frameworks are simply that. It is up to you to put your own stamp on them, to adjust them to suit your purposes so they are used effectively for your purpose. Ultimately, there is no one right way of reflecting, in the same way that there is usually more than one way of doing most things. The frameworks presented in this chapter will provide you with a range of strategies to help you to look beyond your usual ways of thinking and operating and they give you liberating and broadening perspectives on the ways you experience life.

Many models and frameworks for reflection exist, and of necessity I have chosen to present and explore three of these in detail. These are used most commonly, both in educational experiences and in the literature, and can be

Seminal
Important,
influencing later
developments

seen as *seminal* theories that underpin much of reflective practice foundational perspectives. However, I hope these will whet your appetite to explore further and really expand the strategies that you use to learn from and develop your practice. It may be that for coursework purposes you are restricted to those provided by your lecturers. However, this does not stop you experimenting in the work you do by yourself – in your reflective journal or personal critical reflection work and reflective reviews, for instance. Perhaps you could try new strategies working with your mentors and supervisors in practice? They may be familiar with a larger range of frameworks that they can introduce you to and help you explore.

USING GOODMAN'S LEVELS OF REFLECTION

Goodman's levels of reflection were briefly introduced in Chapter 1. This chapter develops these further to show how you will gradually increase the depth and breadth of your reflective work through your course.

First level reflection

When you begin your reflective practice you will only be expected to be working at Goodman's first level (Goodman, 1984). This expects your work to be largely descriptive, where you concentrate on getting down the basic facts of what happened and show some awareness of what was going on at the time. Goodman suggests that at this level you will be reflecting in order to reach given objectives. These can be seen as relating to efficiency, effectiveness and accountability for one's actions.

The first step in reflective practice
is describing what happened.

Sometimes these accounts will read more as a story than as a piece of academic work. However, your assessor/supervisor will only be looking for evidence that you can identify the features of the incident you are describing and that you have learned something from it as a result. An example of this is given in the following case study.

Case study

First level reflection

Sharifa is aged 22 years and at the beginning of the second year as an Adult field nursing student. She lives at home with her parents and two elder sisters, together with their husbands. She has rarely experienced working with male patients, and, as a practicing Muslim, does not socialize with men outside of the family.

"I arrived on the ward at 7.30 am ready to begin a day shift. After receiving handover, my mentor assigned me the job of aiding Chris to have a shower with the help of a health care assistant. Chris is well-known to the staff on the ward as he has end-stage AIDS and has received his in-patient antiretroviral therapy here. He is not expected to live until Christmas, even though he is only 29-years old. He is mentally competent but is physically unable to manage many basic physical self-care activities such as his hygiene due to extreme fatigue, breathlessness and needing to manage an oxygen cylinder. He is largely bed, wheelchair or chair-bound, but can manage to move between the two with support. He is unsafe on his feet so mobilizes with a walking frame when able to walk. Usually, his long-term civil partner, David, helps with all personal care, but was unable to be on the ward today.

I approached Chris's bed and asked his consent to take him to the bathroom. Although used to carers helping him shower, he looked rather nervous – I think it was because he was having two young female nurses caring for his personal needs. As David usually cares for him, he must have felt a little uncomfortable, particularly as he is now physically emaciated. At the thought of myself being in his position and being a similar age as him, I began to feel embarrassed too.

I thought that I could not possibly be a professional individual if I let my embarrassment and sympathy get in the way of my nursing care.

We assisted Chris to shower and needed to help him wash as he was so exhausted. I knew he was uncomfortable and wanted to be able to wash himself, but was unable to do so. I was finding it difficult to look him in the eye, especially when it came to washing his genitalia, because at this stage he was getting increasingly embarrassed. I tried to ease this by making conversation, but in a way this made things worse because I felt I was being patronizing in what I was saying. Although physically he requires help, his mind is still fully active.

Afterwards we dried Chris, dressed him and returned him in the wheelchair to bed. To the health care assistant it was another job done, but the feelings of embarrassment I had afterwards, as I am sure was the case with Chris, stayed with me for some time. I realize that I need to overcome my reticence with men as I cannot choose the patients I work with on the basis of their gender. However, this was a particularly difficult experience for me as I am not used to male nudity and find conversing with men challenging, let alone giving intimate physical care."

This example presents a good descriptive account of both what happened and Sharifa's part in it. She incorporates her feelings about what was happening at the time, but does not go much beyond this, other than in equating her feelings with the patient's and thinking a little about her role of a nurse in relation to her religious and cultural background. In this way she achieves her objectives in exploring her reaction to the experience. She identifies her efficiency, in that the task was achieved. She questions whether she was really effective as a nurse because, although the shower itself was completed, she felt she had not addressed Chris's psychological and emotional needs. She recognizes her accountability as a student nurse and sees this as being more than that expected from a support worker.

Reflective accounts at this level may be used as the basis for discussion with your supervisor, or perhaps in a classroom situation with your colleagues. You may also start to build a bank of these in a portfolio as evidence of your beginning work as a reflective practitioner. But, as you get further on in your course, you will be expected to become more analytical in this kind of work and start to present conclusions. This is where you will move to Goodman's second level.

Second level reflection

At this level, you will be starting to identify your learning and drawing conclusions about patient care that are transferable to other situations. You will be using theoretical concepts to explore and explain what has happened, and to provide you with further insight and understanding. In short, you will be creating your own knowledge base by applying theory to practice, and considering theory in the light of practice. Goodman suggests that reflection at this level shows awareness of the implications of both personal and professional values in addition to identifying the rationale and evidence basis of actions taken.

An example of reflection at this level is shown in the case study below.

Case study

Second level reflection

Shonagh is a third year Adult field nursing student from Ireland, aged 38 years.

"Mrs James had been admitted to the ward following a fall at home and had multiple bruising and cuts to her body. Throughout her time on the ward she had been mildly confused, with a tendency to wander unsupervised. As Oleveczky (2009) states, this is a major concern within hospitals and care facilities, as falls account for 70 per cent of all inpa-

tient accidents, with 60 per cent in patients over 70 years of age resulting in moderate to severe injuries. We were told that Mrs James was unsteady on her feet and should not attempt to walk on her own without assistance.

On the day this event happened, we noticed that Mrs James was particularly agitated. This could have been a behavioural cue that she was in pain. We asked her the problem, and administered analgesics when she confirmed our suspicions that she was in pain. She settled back onto her bed. Shortly after this she rang the call bell and told me of her continuing discomfort, wanting further pain relief. I explained that the tablets she had been given would take some time to take effect and that she should stay on her bed as they might make her drowsy and likely to fall (Rhalimi *et al.*, 2009). As Desbien and Wu (2000, cited by Husband 2002) suggest, I was aware that elderly patients often pay little regard to the side effects associated with pain relief.

I began to walk away, but was called back by Mrs James. I felt slightly annoyed, because of the time I had taken in explaining the situation to her. However, as I turned to respond, Mrs James fell to the floor as she tried to get out of bed again, hitting her face heavily.

Initially I froze with the shock of seeing her falling, and then I felt panic about what I should be doing. This was the first time I had witnessed a patient falling and because of my lack of medical knowledge and inexperience I was scared by it and did not know what to do. I called for help.

My inclination was to help Mrs James to her feet, but the staff nurse said to leave her where she was as she might have further injuries. I have found since that over 30 per cent of patients aged 65 and over experience at least one serious fall each year costing the NHS more than £4.6m per day (BBC, 2010). Eighty-four per cent of these accidents occur in an acute care setting.

This incident has helped me to draw understanding from the situation. While I felt guilty initially because I felt the incident was my fault, as Anderson (2008) says, whilst up to 30 per cent of falls are preventable, and falls that do occur often result from known predictors, the remainder are not. Reflecting on this incident has enabled me to develop my understanding of ways of minimizing falls in the elderly, and prepared me to respond effectively and correctly if they do. My primary objective is to be armed with the knowledge of what to do, so that I can respond more quickly. I need to be more effective at communicating with confused patients. I also need to understand more about risk assessment, which aims to establish the levels of care required, along with areas of caution, and can be seen as fundamental to all patient care" (Kim and Hood, 2001).

References

Anderson, K.E. (2008) Falls in the elderly. *Journal of the. Royal College of Physicians of Edinburgh* **38** (1) 38–43 http://www.bbc.co.uk/news/10353642

Husband, L. (2002) Caring for the patient in pain, in *Common Foundation Studies in Nursing*, 3rd edn (eds N. Kenworthy, G. Snowley and C. Gilling). Churchill Livingstone, Edinburgh, pp. 457–480.

Kim, S. and Hood, K. (2001) A falls risk-assessment tool in an elderly care environment. *British Journal of Nursing*, **10**, 440–449.

Olveczky, D. (2009) How do I keep my elderly patients from falling? *The Hospitalist* September. http://www. the-hospitalist.org/details/article/327725

Rhalimi, M., Helou, R., Jaecker, P. (2009) Medication use and increased risk of falls in hospitalized elderly patients: a retrospective, case control. *Drugs Aging* **26** (10) 84–52

Shonagh shows how her experience has triggered a need to go and develop his understanding through reading. In turn, but this is reflected back into practice as she develops her action plan for what she can do should she meet the situation again. She is moving confidently between theory and practice here so that her actions are underpinned by her knowledge. Shonagh also demonstrates the beginnings of her awareness of her role as a professional practitioner, bound by personal and professional beliefs of what role a nurse should take. She was concerned that this accident occurred while the patient was under her care. She identified a knowledge deficit and wanted to ensure that she had the understanding to prevent harm occurring in future. Shonagh is clearly demonstrating the ability to transfer her learning from this one case out to general principles for dealing with similar situations.

Third level reflection

Finally, Goodman's third level includes an acknowledgement of the wider influences of ethical and political influences on care delivery. This takes the reflective activity one stage further by relating the parameters of care to societal norms and constraints, such as health policy, health economics and resources. The following case study illustrates how a lack of resources can inhibit optimum care.

Third level reflection

Lizzie is a third year occupational therapy student working a placement with the OT in the local social services department. She is approaching qualification and is therefore able to make visits by herself but always discusses these in detail in clinical supervision with her supervisor the same, or following, day.

"Having assessed Mr Sheppard's mobility at home I returned to the office to place the order for grab rails to be put in his bathroom and for a stair lift to get him upstairs. There was no possibility of moving the bed downstairs because of the room available.

I am so frustrated!

Here is a man blocking a much-needed elderly care bed who cannot go home because of a lack of resources to supply and fit simple mobility aids. We have the grab rails, but fitting will be delayed for a month because of a lack of carpenters at Social Services. The chair lift is out of the question until after April (six months away) because the budget for such things has already been spent. The couple are unable to afford a lift themselves and they are reluctant to go to charities for help.

I am beginning to understand far more fully the role that OTs play in the multidisciplinary team, and how crucial they are to enabling patients to be discharged, particularly when delayed discharge is such a major cause of 'bed-blocking' in the NHS at present.

A week later Having followed this incident further I have come to an understanding of the situation. We do not live in a society where everything is free and available on demand, although this is often the impression that we get. Social Services have a budget allocated to home aids and resourcing their fitting. There is no more money available for this once the budget has been allocated. They have only two carpenters and one is on long-term sick leave, so the waiting list for fitting grab rails is necessarily long. So, what are the alternatives? I talked to Mr and Mrs Sheppard about re-arranging downstairs so that a single bed can be brought into the living room, and they have got their son-in-law to do this. The room has been made safe by removing slip rugs and clutter from the floor, and trailing leads. The lighting has been improved with spotlights and higher-voltage bulbs. As Mrs Sheppard is the principal carer, and physically sound, we have decided to ask the Red Cross to provide a commode that she can empty in the bathroom upstairs. I have talked with the GP about care help for washing and bathing so that Mrs Sheppard can have a break. Mr Sheppard will be going home in a couple of days – three weeks earlier than would have been possible if we had waited for the rails to be fitted.

This is not an ideal solution, but is the best possible given the circumstances."

This excerpt omits the theoretical exploration and justification that was present in the original in order to illustrate the third-level criteria of considering the political and social context of care.

Lizzie had assumed that resources are unlimited and were available dependent on need. This was an extremely valuable lesson for her, as she not only found alternatives to the problem that were workable and practical, she also realized early in her career that care is not value-free but is dependent upon societal values and priorities, which may not be in the interests of every individual.

Reflective activity

Think about the reflective work that you have already done – whether as part of your course, as a result of completing activities from this book or in other parts of your life. Which levels of reflection have you been working at? What would you need to do to move to the next level(s)?

KEY POINTS

- Goodman's definitions of the levels of reflection provide a useful way of understanding the different levels at which we reflect
- They may be equated with academic levels in our courses
- Reflective practitioners need to work towards reaching Goodman's third level

All levels can be used in any of the strategies and frameworks for reflection that you will use. Three frameworks are now worked through, illustrated with case studies, to help you explore and understand how structures can help you in beginning your reflective practice.

GIBBS'S REFLECTIVE CYCLE

The first framework explored has been developed from Kolb's ideas in educational theory and develops the features of the ERA cycle. This is the reflective cycle developed by Graham Gibbs (1988) and is shown in Figure 3.1.

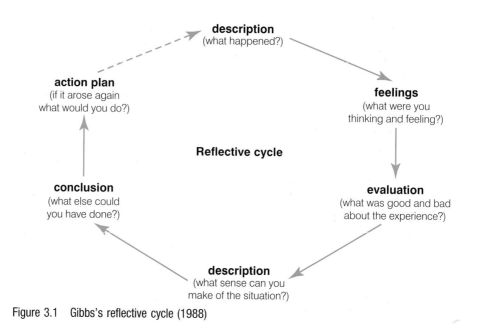

Figure 3.1   Gibbs's reflective cycle (1988)

Gibbs's framework has achieved the status of a seminal theory in reflective practice in health care and it would be difficult to find any paper or textbook on reflective practice written in the past 15 years that did not draw on his work in some way. Gibbs's cycle consists of six stages that guide you through the stages of the reflective process by asking a series of cue questions. Prior to this, the critical incident to be reflected on must have been chosen (see Chapter 1).

Stage 1: Description of the event

The starting point is to write down, or tell someone else, a short version of the event you want to reflect on. The type of event you select will depend on whether you want to share this with someone else or whether, at this time, you need to keep it to yourself. At this stage, it is important to get as much down about the event as you can in an objective way. Some of the things that you might include (using the six wise men) are:

- *Where* were you and *why*?
- *What* happened?
- *When* did it happen?
- *Who* else was there?
- *What* were you doing?
- *What* were the other people doing?
- *What* was your part in this?
- *What* parts did the other people play?
- *How* did you react?
- *What* was the result?

Stage 2: Feelings

At this stage you try to recall, and explore, the things that were going on inside your head during the event. These are often the things that cause us to feel happy, or dissatisfied with the event, and why it sticks in our mind in the first place. This is also the stage which you might find difficult to share with other people. Some questions that are useful here are:

- How were you feeling when the event started?
- What were you thinking at the time?
- What were you thinking about when it happened? How did it make you feel then?
- What did other people's actions/words make you think?
- What did these make you feel?
- How did you feel about the outcome of the event?
- What do you think about it now?
- List the emotions that you have gone through from the start to the finish of the event
- Which of these is most significant or important to you?

Stage 3: Evaluation

When we evaluate something we give it a value, or measure it against some sort of a standard. What we are trying to do is to arrive at some sort of judgement about what has happened so that we can recognize all of its components, and not just those that are at the front of our minds when we think of it. So, the sorts of question that we might ask here are:

- What was good about the experience?
- What was bad about the experience, or didn't go so well?

> **Evaluation**
> Assessing the worth or value of something, to measure it against a standard

Stage 4: Analysis

This means 'to break things down into their component parts' so that they can be explored separately. So we need to ask more detailed questions about the answers to the last stage. We might ask such questions as:

- What went well?
- What did I do well?
- What did others do well?
- What went wrong, or did not turn out the way I thought it should? In what ways did I contribute to this?
- What knowledge/skills/experience did I use/am I lacking?

- Were there any alternative courses of action that I could have taken?
- In what ways did others contribute to this?
- Why might these things have happened?

Stage 5: Conclusion

This differs from the evaluation stage in that now you have explored the issue from different angles and have a great deal more information on which to base your judgement. It is here that you are likely to develop insight into your own and other people's behaviour in terms of how they contributed to the outcome of the event. Sometimes this is difficult, because we may realize that the way we handled an event, or our part in it, might not have been the most effective way of going about things. This, however, is exactly the point! Remember, the purpose of reflection is to learn from experience. Without the detailed analysis and honest exploration that occurs during these stages, it is unlikely that all aspects of the event will be taken into account, and therefore valuable opportunities for learning can be missed. Gibbs suggests that we ask ourselves what we could have done differently as part of this stage.

Stage 6: Action plan

At this stage you are invited to think yourself forward into encountering the event again, and to plan what you would do – would you act differently, or would you be likely to do the same again?

Gibbs' cycle stops here, with anticipated action. The cycle is completed tentatively by suggesting that the next time the event occurs it will be the focus of another reflective cycle. This whole cycle is illustrated in the case study below.

Case study

Parvinder

A student physiotherapist of Asian background, aged 21 in her third year.

Description – what happened? "I had been asked by my supervisor to work with Mrs Singh, an 83-year-old lady in hospital for respite care to give her daughter a break from the day-to-day caring routine. Despite her senile dementia, it was hoped that we would be able to increase her mobility and self-care activities so that she wasn't such a physical drain on her daughter. I was hoping to do some passive stretching exercises with her, before getting her walking with her frame. My supervisor, Casey, was working with other patients on the ward, doing pre-op breathing exercises.

Mrs Singh was with three other patients grouped together at the far end of a Nightingale-type ward and separated from the other patients, who were predominantly recovering from surgery. I had worked with all four patients before and had no worries as I approached Mrs Singh, although I had been on the receiving end of her extensive foul and abusive language before. Mrs Singh presented all members of the caring team with challenges every day, as even the most simple of tasks, such as getting out of bed and taking medicines, were met with refusal, swearing and insulting behaviour – a feature of dementia.

That morning, Mrs Singh was dressed and sitting on a chair beside her bed. I drew the curtains around the bedspace, and positioned everything ready to help her back on to the bed so that we could do some exercises. I was talking to her all the time whilst I was getting ready, but got no verbal response at all. As I bent down to support her in standing up, I felt a sudden sharp scrape down the side of my face. Mrs Singh began to swear quite loudly at me and I was worried that the other patients and staff would hear the shouting and wonder what was going on. I tried to reassure her, but she scratched me again, pulling her nails down the side of my cheek. I was really shocked and, never having been physically attacked before, my first thoughts were to get someone else to help. I ensured Mrs Singh was safely in her chair, drew back the curtains and went to find help."

Feelings – what were you thinking and feeling?

"Initially, my feelings at the time were for Mrs Singh as I was concerned that my actions had caused her to feel threatened and strike out to defend herself. I felt guilty, but stayed calm and tried to think what I had done wrong. I felt embarrassed but Casey was very supportive and reassured me that it wasn't my fault. A few minutes later though I felt very cold and started shaking. I found it difficult that someone I was trying to help would attack me."

Evaluation – what was good and bad about the experience?

"I had prepared for the therapy session with Mrs Singh by reviewing her physio records, and reading the nursing notes when I got to the ward. I had also talked to the Staff Nurse looking after her that morning to find out how she was and whether there had been anything happening that might affect my work with her. Nothing indicated that Mrs Singh was in an aggressive mood that morning. I had also planned what I was going to do in advance. I made sure that I introduced myself, and talked all the time to Mrs Singh, telling her in advance about what I was doing and what the plans were. I drew the curtains to ensure privacy for the transfer to the bed and the exercises.

What was bad was that I was sworn at and ended up getting scratched on my face. As a result I had to go to Occupational Health and have the wound cleaned properly and a tetanus update, then I went home as I was still shocked, so I missed the rest of my clinical experience that day, which I was looking forward to.

I was working by myself at the end of the ward, in a section divided off by a solid division, and thus was out of immediate hearing of the other staff. I also attempted to transfer Mrs Singh by myself."

Analysis – what sense can you make of the situation?

"The result was that we decided not to proceed with the physio that day, so I felt guilty and upset that my actions resulted in the patient not being treated. I felt a failure that I wasn't able to do the job I was expected to do, and as a result the patient suffered. However, Mrs Singh had no recollection of what she had done to me, because of her dementia, and perhaps this was a good thing as it meant that I could go back into her room the next day to continue her therapy. I realized that she hadn't deliberately meant to hurt me, but that this kind of aggressive behaviour is a result of the dementia and was a way of her protecting herself when she felt threatened. Since the incident I have read more about confusion, aggression and dementia, and realize that it always has to be anticipated in patients of this kind, especially when they are not in their familiar environment. I have also suggested to the University that we have some sessions included early in our training about defusing a potentially violent situation, self-defence and breakaway techniques. It would be useful to explore the psychology of being attacked and ways in which we can deal with it and come to terms with it.

I realized that my reactions later, after I had made sure she was safe, were symptoms of shock. I felt very vulnerable and at risk myself, but understand now, after talking it through with Casey, that this is a normal reaction designed to enable us to cope with stressful situations."

Conclusion – what else could you have done? "I realize now that there wasn't a lot that I could have done in that situation, and perhaps the best thing was to leave Mrs Singh to calm down. I did wonder whether I could have done something else in that position and what other choices I had in trying to do what I was supposed to do. I could have stayed with Mrs Singh and tried to calm her down, but I didn't have the knowledge or experience for dealing with aggressive patients, and didn't know what to do.

I wonder though, whether it is really a good idea to work with anyone who has a history of aggressive behaviour by yourself. I also feel that I should have spent longer sitting and talking with her before trying to move her, to get her used to me and create a calm atmosphere. She hadn't said a word to me before I tried to move her, and maybe I ought to have taken a cue from this that she wasn't feeling very co-operative."

Action plan – what would you do if this situation arose again? "I am now more prepared for patients to be violent. I had always thought before that it wouldn't happen to me, and that the person who was attacked was to blame in some way. I don't think that now. In future, where I know that patients have an aggressive history, or even with demented patients, I will be more on my guard. I will take the time to reassure and talk to the patient and ensure that I get their cooperation. I will also try to avoid working alone in an area or where there are patients who can be aggressive."

Reflections on writing the critical incident "While writing this assignment I have been able to re-examine my critical incident properly with adequate time to reflect on every detail of what happened. I have had the opportunity to learn from my mistakes and this will enable me to improve my future patient care and think more about my own safety. Although I concluded that this incident was a negative one, now, on reflection, I see that it was very valuable, especially happening when it did in my course, as I am much more aware of the potential for aggression and violence from patients. This is because I have learned not only about violent patients but also how to use the technique of reflection to help me get through, and understand, what happens in clinical situations. Gibbs's reflective cycle suited this situation because it helped me to break it down and really think about it in a different way. While I hope that I never get attacked again, I do feel that I am more aware of the potential for aggression and have learned to approach situations in a different way from the more naïve attitude that I had before this happened. I have also been prompted to read more about aggression in the NHS, and learn strategies to deal with it. I wouldn't have done this if it hadn't happened to me personally."

Parvinder's use of Gibbs's cycle enabled her both to see the situation in a different way and to learn for the future. This was obviously a very distressing incident for Parvinder, in which she questioned her own actions with a patient and had to face up to her own vulnerability in a situation where she was trying to help. Although the experience itself was negative, the use of Gibbs's cycle enabled her to see the incident in a different way and turn it into a learning experience.

Reflective activity

The only way to really understand this reflective cycle is to use it yourself to explore something that has happened to you recently. We suggest that you use the questions given at each stage to work your way through an event that has stuck in your mind for some reason. You could choose something arising during your course, or your practical placement, or even something like returning faulty goods to a store or having a conversation with a friend about a problem they have. It is useful to write your reflections down at this stage, especially if you are using an event at work as the focus, as you may be able to use it as part of your portfolio or for some other purpose in your course.

Once you have done that, take a few minutes to think about how you felt doing the exercise, using the questions below.

- How useful did you find Gibbs's cycle?
- How easy was it to use?
- Did you have any difficulties using it?
- Did it enable you to see the event from a wider perspective?
- Did it enable you to reach alternative conclusions about the event to the ones you had when you started out?
- How comfortable did you feeling using it?
- Would you choose to use it again?

Try to give the reasons for your answers to these questions.

Gibbs's approach is characteristic of all the strategies, or frameworks, for reflection that have been developed over the succeeding years. Where Gibbs's reflective cycle stops, however, is at the action planning stage, and this is why we have used a broken line to link it back up to the descriptive stage (Figure 3.1). What Gibbs has created is a very good framework for the reflective process, i.e. learning from reflecting on something. But it stops at the stage of proposing action. Hence, the reflection can stop, quite legitimately from this point of view, at predicting action in terms of 'If I encountered the situation again, what would I do differently?' Of course, as anyone with even minimal practice experience knows, it is extremely unlikely that another situation will occur that is exactly the same as an experience that you have already had. Experiences may be similar, but they will not be the same. So, although Gibbs provides us with a useful framework for reflecting in the abstract, and usually away from the scene of practice, he does not provide us with the means to close the cycle, nor to move to reflective practice in terms of taking action.

Part of the reason for this lies in the fact that Gibbs's framework arose from an education context, as opposed to a practice basis.

To move from a framework of theoretical reflection to one that arises from a practice environment, which is likely to be more useful in clinical contexts, the work of Chris Johns is now considered.

JOHNS' MODEL OF STRUCTURED REFLECTION

Chris Johns' model, arising from his work in the Burford Nursing Development, has gone through many developments and presentations since the 1994 version (presented in Palmer *et al.*, 1994). It is used here because it is a framework that is easy to use when beginning reflective practice. Updated versions, including more description and development of the concepts, are described in Johns (2006). Johns himself envisaged this model as being used within a process of guided reflection that has three components:

- Using the model of structured reflection
- Supervision
- Diary structure

Johns says that the model:

> *consists of a series of questions which aim to tune the practitioner into her experience in a structured and meaningful way. It emerged as a natural sequence through which practitioners explored their experiences in supervision.*

> *Johns 1994, cited in Palmer et al., 1994, p. 112*

The framework is presented in Figure 3.2.

The focus for Johns, in developing this framework, was about uncovering and making explicit the knowledge that we use in our practice. So, the framework takes this as its core question, which is explored through the five cue questions. These are further divided into more focused questions to promote detailed reflection. The first two stages of this framework are similar to those already considered.

Core question **What information do I need to access in order to learn through this experience?**

Cue questions

1. Description of the experience

- Phenomenon – describe the here and now experience
- Causal – what essential factors contributed to this experience?
- Context – what are the significant background factors to this experience?
- Clarifying – what are the key processes (for reflection) in this experience?

2. Reflection

- What was I trying to achieve?
- Why did I intervene as I did?
- What were the consequences of my actions for:
  - Myself?
  - The patient/family?
  - The people I work with?
- How did I feel about this experience when it was happening?
- How did the patient feel about it?
- How do I know how the patient felt about it?

3. Influencing factors

- What internal factors influenced my decision making?
- What external factors influenced my decision making?
- What sources of knowledge did/should have influenced my decision making?

4. Could I have dealt with the situation better?

- What other choices did I have?
- What would be the consequences of these choices?

5. Learning

- How do I feel now about this experience?
- How have I made sense of this experience in light of past experiences and future practice?
- How has this experience changed my ways of knowing:
  - Empirics
  - Aesthetics
  - Ethics
  - Personal

Figure 3.2   John's model of structured reflection (Palmer *et al.*, 1994)

Cue question 1: Description of the experience

At the descriptive stage, Johns provides four cue questions to help structure the description of what has happened. These identify:

- The 'phenomenon' or the experience itself
- The cause of the experience

- The context within which it happened, or the background to it
- 'Clarifying' – at this stage the person is asked to 'put the experience back together and look at it as a whole, identifying the key processes occurring within the experience' (Johns, 1994, cited in Palmer *et al.*, 1994, p. 113).

As with other frameworks, this sets the scene and provides the baseline for the rest of the reflection. Where it is being used within a supervisory relationship, or for reflecting with other people, it provides an outline of the experience that the other person can understand and work from.

Johns later dropped the four sub-questions that structure the description of the experience, because he felt they 'interfered with practitioners telling their stories' (Johns, 1998). However, these can be useful for students and practitioners beginning reflection because they help to provide a structure for describing the experience that you might find difficult to do without. Once you become familiar and comfortable with the ways in which you describe your own experiences you may decide that these are no longer necessary.

Cue question 2: Reflection

At this stage Johns' framework enters the analytical stages, asking the familiar questions about what the person did and felt and what the consequences of the actions and feelings were, and attempts to get them to take the role of the other person in predicting/anticipating their responses.

A difference between Gibbs's and Johns' frameworks here is the question that Johns asks in trying to identify what the person was trying to achieve within the event/incident. This is very important, because it relates to that idea of practicality and context that is missing from Gibbs's framework. We rarely enter a clinical situation without first considering what our intentions are and what we want the results to be. Having already decided on these, we tend to plan our actions to achieve these. Even when we are reflecting on 'on-the-spot' decisions and reactions to things that happen to us, we still fast-track forward in our heads to try to achieve some aim that we can predict. As a result of this, we have something to measure our success (or failure) against, and it is this that creates our sense of satisfaction or dissatisfaction.

 Over to you

Look back at Parvinder's story in the previous case study. As a practitioner, she certainly had specific aims in mind when she entered her encounter with Mrs Singh. Can you identify what these might have been?

What was it that caused Parvinder to be so unhappy with what had happened?

In asking this question, 'What were you trying to achieve within the event/incident?'. Johns enables us to identify where the outcomes of an experience do not match up with our intentions. In a clinical situation this is clearly very important, as it enables us to evaluate our performance as practitioners and recognize where we are not achieving what we want to achieve.

Johns also introduces the roles that others have played in the experience at this stage in a more detailed way. Gibbs tends to focus solely on the individual reflecting. For the purposes of this book, 'other people' have been introduced into the cue questions in Gibbs's framework to help you understand further. They are not included in Gibbs's original framework. Johns, however, sees the roles and feelings of others as key to understanding the experience in context. He asks us to think about how the patient was feeling. This can be expanded into identifying how all the other people involved may have been feeling. For instance, there may have been family members, friends or carers with the patient, or other health care professionals or colleagues involved in the incident. It is important for us to try to take the feelings of others into account when exploring how situations occurred, as we can develop a great deal of insight by considering alternative ways of seeing and experiencing things.

However, there is one word of caution here. Johns does go on to ask us how we know what those other people were feeling. This is a reminder that our perceptions of things may not reflect what the other people were actually feeling. So it is probably useful to explore why we think people were feeling the way we think they were, and checking this out. Many things happen as a result of mistaken perceptions and misunderstandings, so we need to work on recognizing where we are making assumptions and where we have evidence to support our conclusions.

Over to you

What assumptions was Parvinder making about how Mrs Singh was feeling during the incident as a result of it? What was she basing these on?

Do you think she was right?

What other explanations can you think of?

This point, of course, applies to anyone who is involved in an incident that you are reflecting on.

Reflective activity

Can you think of an example of your own where you made assumptions about what someone else was thinking and then later found you were wrong?

- What was the situation?
- What assumptions were you making?
- Why did you make these?
- Did you check them out with the other person?
- What did you do on the basis of these assumptions?
- What were the consequences?
- Were these as you expected – if not why not?
- What did you learn as a result of this?

Cue question 3: Influencing factors

Johns specifically asks you to identify the factors that influenced you within the incident. This cue question uses the analytical and interpretive reflective processes. Here you will be trawling back through your previous knowledge, skills and experience to identify the basis on which you made your decisions and the external factors that may also have had some effect on you.

Internal factors are those that arise from yourself – your previous experiences, any similar cases or situations that you have encountered, intuition, etc.

External factors include any knowledge or information that comes from outside of you – the more objective sources, for instance, such as your reading, guidance from your professional bodies, government policy or your employer's procedures and policies.

This is a useful division for the beginning reflector, because it helps us to separate out what it is we know for ourselves as opposed to what comes from outside of us. It is worth remembering, though, that it could be said that anything that we know is actually part of us because we have taken it in and perceived it in a way that is unique to us. Although the source of the knowledge may be external, therefore, our use and transformation of it is in many ways unique. The purpose of reflection here then, is to 'unpack' these influences in order to understand, and perhaps challenge, our way of perceiving the world through identifying and acknowledging just what these influences are.

Each of us is influenced by both
internal and external factors.

Cue question 4: Could I have dealt better with the situation?

This stage involves the reflective process of exploring alternatives. Johns'
phrasing here assumes that the critical incident being explored was one that
could have had a better outcome – it may even have been negative in some
way. In later versions of the framework this has changed, as he comes to
focus more on how we know what we know, rather than on reflection as a
way of changing what we do. Hence, it may be more positive to revert to our
phrasing of 'exploring alternatives' here, as a way of widening our perceptions of how we can deal with situations rather than resting with self-
criticism and self-improvement.

Cue question 5: Learning

Finally, Johns asks us, on the basis of the insights gained during the previous
stages, to identify what we have learned. He asks us how we now feel about
the experience.

Pete's story presents an incident critical for him, that arose on his first day
in placement as a student nurse. It presents a good example of the use of
Johns' framework to this stage of the last cue question. Read this now, and
then take some time to answer the questions that follow it.

Case study

Pete

An 18-year-old adult field student nurse has just started his first work placement.

Describing the phenomenon   "My first placement was on a ward specializing in the surgical care of cardiac patients. Mr Chen, a 68-year-old Chinese man, had previously undergone a triple coronary bypass. During the process various drains and catheters, including a central line and chest drain, had been inserted to assist drug administration to and fluid removal from the thoracic cavity. It had been three days since Mr Chen's operation; his central line had already been removed but his chest drain was still to be taken out. As a student new to the ward, I was not allowed to do this myself but I was to observe the two staff nurses carry out the procedure.

Mr Chen had been tachycardic (raised heart rate) since his operation, setting off the alarm on the cardiac monitor. Although his raised heart rate was not of concern to the staff, and this had been communicated to Mr Chen, the constant noise coming from the monitor was making him very anxious, and it is possible that, given that English is not his first language, he had difficulty understanding the cause of the problem. . He started to have anxiety attacks, began to cry and get in an agitated state, increasing his heart and respiration rates even more. His wife and daughter were unable to be with him to give some support because they had to be at work.

The chest drain was about to be removed but Mr Chen's emotional state created a problem because of his fast breathing and inability to concentrate on what was being said to him. The nurses needed his co-operation in the removal of the drain, but he was too frightened.

As I was not taking part in the procedure, I took it upon myself to calm him down. I sat beside him and held his hand, encouraging him to talk to me in order to take his mind off what was going to happen to him. I told him that removing the drain was the last procedure he would have to undergo and that, although he felt worried, once it was removed he would feel much more comfortable. I also told him that I would be with him through the whole procedure and that it would be over very quickly. I could see that I was having a positive effect on him as his breathing slowed down and he ceased crying. I continued to talk to him and reassured him that the two qualified nurses and I would take care of him. Mr Chen was soon calm enough to concentrate on his breathing, the chest drain was then swiftly out and a dressing was applied to the wound.

Having not been on a ward before, this was my first major interaction with a patient, and the two nurses involved told me I handled the situation well and contributed to the removal of the drain by helping Mr Chen relax, resulting in his respiration rate slowing down."

Reflection   "When seeing the distress experienced by Mr Chen before the procedure I felt unsettled and worried and instinctively felt that I wanted to help him. I realized I was the person to calm him down – although the nurses calmed him slightly themselves, they were concentrating on the procedure so their attention was not fully centred on Mr Chen's emotional state. Therefore, as I wasn't actively taking part in the removal of the drain, I could give all my attention to him.

I thought my actions were justified: the patient needed to be reassured swiftly or the chest drain could not have been removed as quickly and efficiently and his anxiety would have been prolonged.

During the situation I was faced with many thoughts. Initially I wasn't sure if I was helping. I felt as though I was a hindrance and that my observing the patient might have been making him feel more uncomfortable. When he grasped my hand, though, I realized he was happy for me to be there and was looking to me for reassurance. I felt relieved that I was actually helping and contributing to his care, despite my inexperience and lack of knowledge. He seemed gratified to have me beside him, he felt he wasn't alone and looked upon me as a friend as well as part of the nursing team looking after him. After the drain was removed he said that having a familiar and friendly face certainly made a difference, it made him feel confident and as though he was being taken care of. He said that this, for him, was an important part of nursing."

Influencing factors
"Many internal and external factors influenced my actions. Seeing people distressed unsettles me. I felt uncomfortable with the idea that Mr Chen was suffering from discomfort and wanted to do something to relieve his anxiety. Not being able to help with the procedure, I felt incompetent and helpless just 'observing'. I wanted to take part in one way or another, and having limited nursing skills I realized this was how I could make my contribution.

With Mr Chen feeling distressed, his heart rate was getting higher and higher, and he was aware of this as he could hear it on the monitor. As I didn't know how to interpret the readings on the monitor correctly, the apparent increase on the monitor was making me anxious too, as I thought something serious might happen. My knowledge of cardiac conditions and treatment was very limited so I panicked and thought the situation was worse than it actually was. This was the reason that I reacted in the way that I did. I had previously read that the therapeutic use of touch helps in many ways, and that it can help to build a rapport between nurse and patient, thus bringing about trust in the relationship. By holding his hand I thought reassurance would be provided to let him know that he was not alone, therefore helping to calm him down. Personal experience also made me think that interaction such as kind words and attention between individuals can help relieve a stressful situation."

Alternative actions
"After the nurses and I had finished working with Mr Chen, I didn't think too much about what had happened and wasn't convinced that I had played any role in caring for him. As far as I was concerned, I didn't actually 'do' anything beneficial for the situation. I thought this until one of the staff nurses involved in the procedure, who happened to be my mentor, highlighted to me that I had performed some nursing care with a positive outcome for the patient. Although I didn't physically take part, I successfully supported the patient emotionally through what for him was an emotionally distressing experience."

Learning
"I look back now and realize that I underestimated the use of 'basic' nursing care and that patients' feelings and emotions are equally as important as the reason for their hospitalization. I now believe that in order for me to become a good nurse in future practice, and to provide holistic care, basic nursing skills have to be learned, before concentrating on the more 'in depth' side of nursing such as medical procedures, treatment and diagnosis.

Having not worked in a nursing environment before, I have no experience to compare this incident to; however, I feel that I have learned a great deal from working with Mr Chen and the nurses involved. Although in this case my feelings of panic were not detected, I have learned that many patients in the future will consider me to be the professional and will expect me to be in control in any situation. A nurse showing panic may unsettle a patient, resulting in lack of confidence and trust.

This, in turn, is likely to affect the treatment being given.

As a student with limited experience, I realize that as my course progresses I will become more confident in dealing with situations of this nature. However, increasing my knowledge of some common medical procedures will assist me in future clinical practice as it helps me to understand some of the problems that I may be faced with when implementing treatments."

Reflections on the use of the framework
"By using Johns' reflective model as a guide, I have been able to reflect on the incident and this has enabled me to evaluate the actions that I took during the incident, questioning whether my response was appropriate. It has also allowed me to think of other ways I could have dealt

with the situation and the possible outcomes. The reflective strategy has helped me to learn from this experience and has given me an insight into how I might improve my own future practice. It has also shown me that, by continuing the reflective process by following reflective frameworks such as Johns' in future incidents, I may improve the ways of dealing with situations, and acknowledge that I am actually learning something from every experience that I have. The importance of reflection has been reinforced to me in writing up this critical incident, because I hadn't really thought about the importance of emotional support for patients before, nor the effect of putting on a uniform and having patients regard me as a professional."

Over to you

Summarize the learning that Pete has identified from this incident.

- What other learning can you see in this account that he has not identified?
- Why might he not have seen this himself?

If you look closely at Figure 3.2, you will see that Pete has not gone on to complete the final cue question posed by Johns, that of exploring the incident through what he has called 'ways of knowing'. This phrase relates back to the original purpose for his framework, to create a strategy for learning through uncovering the knowledge that we have and identifying what more we need to know in order to practise effectively. Johns is a nurse by background, and therefore has based his model in nursing. However, this provides a useful framework that is easily translated into other health care professions, and therefore warrants further development here.

Johns considers it important to recognize our 'knowing' and has adopted a typology of knowledge identified by Barbara Carper in 1978. She identified four ways of knowing that can be found in nursing and named them:

- Empirics
- Ethics
- Personal
- Aesthetics

Empirics Carper calls this the science of nursing, which emerged as a concept in nursing during the late 1950s. It draws on traditional ideas of science in which reality is viewed as something that can be verified by other observers. Empirics are based on the assumption that what is known is that which is accessible through the senses, i.e. that can be observed and measured in some way. Empirics use the processes of describing, explaining and predicting the phenomena in the world through classic scientific methods. The ideal of scientific theory is that all its major ideas are expressed in terms that can be translated to 'out there' – empiric reality. Very often, theories of nursing, and other health care professions, are seen to be lacking when judged against scientific parameters, and this was certainly the case when Carper was writing. What empirics give to us are the scientific background and theories that inform much of our practice. Examples of empirics that provide us with ways of knowing in health care are: physiological processes and anatomical structure; pharmacology; psychology, etc.

Ethics This incorporates what Carper called 'moral knowledge' or what is believed to be right or wrong in the way that we interact with other people. It includes matters of obligation or what ought to be done in particular situations. It involves making moment-to-moment judgements about what should be done, what is right and what is responsible. This may mean confronting conflicting values, norms, interests or principles in different situations. This is especially relevant for all kinds of professional health care practice, as we are dealing with unique individuals over whom we very often have powers of life or death, and the quality of their lives. Our actions may determine the ways in which people experience their lives, particularly where they are unable to look after themselves, or make decisions that affect their lives – for instance, in the case of elderly people with dementia or people who are unconscious. Ethical knowing requires both an implicit knowing to base on-the-spot decisions on and knowledge of the formal principles and ethical theories of the disciplines. What it cannot do is to describe or predict what a decision should be; rather, it provides insight into what decisions are possible and why. The processes we use within our ethical knowing are those of clarifying, valuing and advocating for others.

Personal Carper sees this as the inner experience of becoming a whole, aware self. She suggests that, through knowing oneself, one is able to know another human being as a person because we have a concept of shared human experience. She says that we cannot reflect personal knowledge; that it is retrospective in that one can only describe the self that was when something was happening.

The processes that we use in personal knowing are:

- Opening (being open to others)
- Centring (focusing on the patient)
- Realizing (understanding the other person through recognizing our own experiences).

Aesthetics Carper sees this as the art of nursing, which involves seeing situations as wholes, not component parts. It is the way that nursing is expressed and made visible through actions, bearing, conduct, attitudes and the interactions of the nurse with her patients. She suggests that aesthetics involve what is possible, not necessarily what is concrete, as we reflect on alternative courses of action.

This way of knowing includes what we learn as a result of our professional experiences. It is how we 'know' how to select from our total knowledge and wealth of experience that we have built up in the past, in order to perform what has been termed by Jacobs-Kramer and Chinn (1988) the 'art-act'. This is very often an unconscious process that we are not aware of unless we stop and think about it. The processes that we use in aesthetics are engaging, interpretation, envisioning.

Carper (1978) said that all four of these are present in all of our interactions, and that it is unlikely that one alone would inform the way that we act. However, they combine in different proportions, depending on what we are doing. While this approach to how we know the things that inform our professional actions arises from nursing, it is possible to use it to explore the ways that other health care professions also use their sources of knowing. This is illustrated in the case study below.

Case study

Nick's experience – considering ways of 'knowing' in a physiotherapy interaction

Nick is a third year physiotherapy student, approaching the end of his degree programme and hoping to work in sports rehabilitation on qualification. He is particularly interested in motivating children to play sport safely, and eventually would like to become a football club physio.

Nick is designing a rehabilitation programme for Mark, aged ten, who injured his knee playing football. He has undergone surgery to the cruciate ligament in his left knee and now needs to work on rebuilding strength and mobility. The ways of knowing that inform his decisions can be broken down into Carper's framework as follows.

Empirics Nick will use the information from his physical assessment of Mark to plan what exercises he will need and to predict a programme for his progress. These arise from his knowledge of anatomy and physiology and of healing processes. He will also draw on his ongoing physiotherapy education experiences, in which he learned a range of therapies and exercises that he can select from to design a programme appropriate to Mark's particular needs and he predicts will be effective.

He will also be taking into account Mark's age and lifestyle, what range of movement he needs to regain and what he will need to be able to do in the future, taking account of his age, and that most of his daily living needs are provided by his family. He also draws on his knowledge of motivational theories from psychology, and works within a cognitive framework of enabling Mark to understand the programme and what he is trying to achieve, so that he is committed to it as the best way forward for him. He engages Mark's mother, father and sister in the programme, knowing that their support and motivation will be key to optimal recovery.

Ethics Nick's professional relationship with Mark is regulated by the Health Profession's Council's *Standards of Conduct, Performance and Ethics* (2004), by law and by the commonly accepted 'rules' of interpersonal relationships. Mark and his family can expect Nick to treat him with respect and civility and to assure him that he has his best interests at heart. He needs to enable Mark and his parents to understand the programme being devised so that he has their informed consent.

Equally, he can expect that they will treat him as a professional in terms of his language, the type of touching that happens between them, and the ways in which they negotiate his programme.

Personal knowing As a human being himself Nick can understand the anxiety and worries that Mark has about his mobility and capacities in the future. Nick is aware that he needs to recover as soon as possible so that he can return to school and interactions with his peer-group – crucial at his stage of development and to his future education. Nick understands that very often Mark's aggressive manner with him is not about him specifically but because of his frustration over his mobility, inability to engage in physical activities with his friends, go to his out-of-school activities, and generally do what boys of ten do! He also knows that being able to play football and being part of a team, is part of who Mark is

and is central to his self-esteem. It helps him to define who he is and is crucial to his self-image. Nick knows this because of how he defines and identifies himself.

Aesthetics As a final year student, Nick has built up a wealth of experience in dealing with sports injuries. He 'knows' how to approach Mark and maintain a positive and motivating attitude because of his experiences, and because patients need to have faith in their therapists. They need to be able to depend on him, as a professional, to keep them going when progress seems slow and they become dejected. He also knows when to stop and pull back, judging how much further Mark can be pushed with reference to his previous experiences with similar patients, and the further training and experience he has had in working with children with sports injuries.

Over to you

Go back to Parvinder's account now, and complete the final stage of Johns's framework. Identify what you think are the components of the four ways of knowing that she has used in this critical incident.

- How do these differ from your answers in the previous exercise?
- How useful do you think this strategy is for helping us to understand what knowledge we are using in situations?

Johns' model of structured reflection can, of course, be used very successfully without the final cue question about identifying our ways of knowing. In fact, it seems to have become the most commonly used framework for reflective activity as it is particularly helpful in having the cue questions. Johns' later versions of the model, however, give more centrality to the four ways of knowing. His version 15, published in 2006, is reproduced in Figure 3.3 to show you the comparison.

Bring the mind home

- Focus on a description that seems significant in some way
- What particular issues seem significant to pay attention to?
- How were others feeling and what made them feel that way?
- How was I feeling and what made me feel that way?
- What was I trying to achieve and did I respond effectively?
- What were the consequences of my actions on the patient, others, myself?
- What factors influenced the way I was feeling, thinking and responding?
- What knowledge did or might have informed me?
- To what extent did I act for the best and in tune with my values?
- How does this situation connect with previous experience?
- How might I respond more effectively given this situation again?
- What would be the consequences of alternative actions for the patient, others and myself?
- What factors might constrain me acting in new ways?
- How do I NOW feel about this experience?
- Am I more able to support myself and others better as a consequence?
- Am I more able to realize desirable practice?

Figure 3.3   Johns' 2006 model of structured reflection, version 15

Reflective activity

Using either of the versions of Johns' model for structured reflection, explore a critical incident that you have had. You could choose to write it down, so that you have a template and a model case constructed for further use. Or, you could choose to use the cue questions for reflecting with another person, maybe a fellow student on your course, or with your supervisor.

It is important, whichever way you choose to do this, to follow this up with some analysis of the framework itself, so you are conscious of the decision making that you are using. Try to answer the following questions:

- How useful did you find Johns' model of structured reflection?
- How easy was it to use?
- Did you have any difficulties using it?
- Did it enable you to see the event from a wider perspective?

- Did it enable you to reach alternative conclusions about the event to the ones you had when you started out?
- Did you identify the knowledge that you were using in the situation?
- How useful is it to be aware of the types of knowing that you are using?
- How comfortable did you feel using it?
- Would you choose to use it again?

Try to give the reasons for your answers to these questions.

KEY POINTS

- As a strategy arising from a practitioner's view point, Johns' model for structured reflection was designed with practitioners' needs in mind.
- Johns incorporates a strategy for recognizing and exploring the knowledge underpinning our practice.
- Johns stops at propositions for action, rather than asking what the practitioner will do.

Johns' framework demonstrates a personal awareness of ourselves, our knowledge and actions. But even in exploring alternatives, it asks what you *could* do rather than what you *will* do, and therefore allows us to stay in the realms of possibility. There is still no link between theoretical and contemplative reflection and the movement from this into action, so it therefore is not really reflective practice as defined in this book. One strategy that does do that, and is starting to be used more extensively in health care practice, is the framework proposed by Borton (1970).

BORTON'S DEVELOPMENTAL FRAMEWORK

Borton's framework presents a relatively simple model that is very suitable for novice practitioners but can be used at different levels as students become more adept at reflecting on their practice, and more critically analytical. It is based on the need of practitioners to operate in the real world of practice – the need to identify, make sense of and respond to real-life situations. It asks the person to reflect using three basic starting points to the questions:

- **What? type questions, such as: What happened? What was I doing? What were others doing?**
  This combines the reflective processes of identifying the experience and describing it in detail.

● **So what? type questions, such as: So what more do I need to know in order to understand the situation? So what could I have done that was different?**

At this stage the student breaks down the situation and tries to make sense of it by analyzing and evaluating in order to draw conclusions. In this way a personal theory about the experience is created that is unique to the individual. He/she may draw on several sources to do this, including their own previous experiences, the knowledge and experience of others and accepted knowledge and theory, such as library sources. Finally, the student has sufficient information and understanding to move to the final stage. This stage combines the processes of *analyzing* and *interpreting* the situation.

● **Now what? type questions, such as: Now what do I need to do to make things better? Now what will I do? Now what might be the consequences of this action?**

At this stage the student plans intervention and action according to the personal theory devised. This stage combines the processes of *exploring alternatives* and *planning action* that will be put into practice. It is significant here that the framework enables the practitioner to consider the possible consequences of different alternative strategies for action. It enables these alternatives to be both considered and evaluated so that action taken is *thoughtful* action.

It is clear here, that the purpose of reflecting is to develop, or change practice. Therefore it does present a framework that bridges the two ERA components of reflective processes and taking action.

The following case study was written by a student biomedical scientist working as part of a team looking at strategies to reduce the incidence of methicillin-resistant *Staphylococcus aureus* (MRSA) in Elderly Care wards. This particular example illustrates the use of reflective practice in problem-solving, as opposed to the previous case study, which is based on a personal experience in care-giving.

Case study

Robert's experience in the laboratory

Robert is a 30-year-old microbiologist with a BSc who is studying for a Masters degree part-time to enable him to become registered as a clinical scientist. He has six years' work experience in his present job.

What? "I work in the microbiology section of a hospital laboratory. I am responsible for overseeing the work of my section, as well as analyzing and interpreting results from samples sent in. My particular specialty is wound swabs.

I had noticed, over a period of a few months, that the vast majority of swabs from elderly inpatients result in MRSA being isolated."

So what? "If extended sensitivity tests are not set up on Day 1 then there is a possible delay in the correct therapy being prescribed. Delays in correct treatment can be catastrophic for the patient concerned and can result in the spread of the organism to other patients. MRSA is becoming endemic in many hospital wards, particularly those for the elderly, and is a severe risk for vulnerable patients. However, the setting up of extra sensitivity tests where not needed, is a waste of laboratory resources."

Now what? "For the benefit of the patient and all others, where *Staphylococcus aureus* is isolated from elderly patients extended sensitivities should be set up on Day 1.

This has now become common practice in the department."

Reflection on the use of the reflective framework "As a microbiologist working in a laboratory where our work is directed by standard operating procedures, I initially found it difficult to conceive of a situation where reflection could be useful. However, when I stepped back and thought about it more, I realized that it is easy to think about our work being simply about bench testing and experiments, and that there is actually a great deal going on beyond the world of the laboratory that influences and affects our work.

The incidence of MRSA in elderly patients had been increasing for months, yet, because the microbiologists had been dealing with the samples on an individual basis, the increase had gone unnoticed. It wasn't until I dealt with several in a row when covering for another member of staff that the penny dropped that there might be a problem here. Borton's framework enabled me to explore the situation rationally by using the cue questions. It is not complicated, and can be used with any type of situation. A more complicated framework would have put me off; many of these ask about feelings and personal action, which, to be quite honest, isn't appropriate in this sort of situation. The simple 'what–so what–now what' framework is easy to carry around in my head and use whenever a problem arises. I have even used it when dealing with other staff in a managerial capacity, and in helping to analyze problems within our multidisciplinary team in the lab."

Many students echo Robert's thoughts about using Borton's framework. Its very simplicity means that it can be carried around in your head and easily remembered. Robert's example demonstrates the use of reflection to identify and solve problems, as opposed to dealing with a critical incident that may have arisen for an individual.

The difference between Borton's approach and Gibbs's and Johns's frameworks is clear in this example too, in that the reflective activity actually led to action being taken, rather than it being proposed or tentative. It moves from the realms of 'maybe' back into the real world of practice.

Borton's framework is being increasingly used by health care professionals as a strategy for reflection, and this has prompted Rolfe (Rolfe *et al.*, 2011) to develop it further in terms of adding in cue questions to flesh out the basic three questions. The expanded version is shown in Figure 3.4.

Descriptive level of reflection	Theory and Knowledge building level of reflection	Action-oriented level of reflection
What	**So what...**	**Now what...**
...is the • problem • difficulty • reason for being stuck • reason for feeling bad • reason we don't get on, etc.? ... was my role in the situation? ... was I trying to achieve? ... action did I take? ... was the response of others? ... were the consequences: • for my patient • for myself • for others? ... feelings did it invoke • in the patients • in myself • in others? ... was good/bad about the experience?	...does this tell me/teach me/imply/mean about: • me • my patient • others • our relationship • my patient's care • the model of care I am using • my attitudes ... was going through my mind as I acted? ... did I base my actions on? ... other knowledge can I bring to the situation? ... could/should I have done to make it better? ... is my new understanding of the situation? ... broader issues arise from the situation?	...do I need to do in order to: • make things better • stop being stuck • improve my patient's care • resolve the situation • feel better • get on better • etc., etc.? ... broader issues need to be considered if this action is to be successful? ... might be the consequences of this action?

Figure 3.4   A framework for reflexive practice (*Rolfe et al.,* 2011)

You will notice that this is called a framework for *reflexive,* as opposed to *reflective practice.* This means that the reflective spiral is created, as the action takes place in order to *change* the experience rather than simply to learn from it. The three key stages identified by Borton are built upon by incorporating the cyclical process described by Gibbs and many of the cue questions proposed by Johns. What makes the framework one for reflexive practice, is that action takes place as a result, and thus the experience is changed, producing a new situation. The reflexive practitioner therefore, is someone who continually practises reflectively, learning from and changing situations continually. This might seem a tall order when you are starting off as a student within a health care profession. But, at some stage you will need to move into this way of practising, as you begin to make the links between the experiences that you have.

Borton's framework is a generic one that can be used by anyone, and indeed, Rolfe (Rolfe *et al.*, 2011) provides two issues to be considered before Borton's framework is adopted, suggesting that active selection is needed. He suggests the following about the Borton's framework:

- He is presenting a framework, not a model, making no claims that it is a representation or description of the process of reflection; it is merely an ordered set of cues through which the practitioner might structure reflective thoughts.

- It is a generic framework that can be employed to structure internal, spoken, or written reflections either alone, with a facilitator, or in a group. Because of this it may not suit individual needs, and the cue questions are therefore intended to be open to change and revision for different practitioners in different situations.

Reflective activity

Try using Borton's framework for yourself. You could choose either the simplified 'what – so what – now what' version, or work through the expanded one proposed by Rolfe.

It is worth taking some time to choose the experience to reflect on.

You could re-work the previous example that you used in the Gibbs or Johns frameworks. If you do this you'll have a comparison of what you learned from both, and be able to evaluate how useful each of them will be to you. Alternatively, you may choose to select a completely different experience or incident.

Work through the different stages to complete the reflective process.

Once you have done that, take a few minutes to evaluate the framework itself.

- How useful did you find Borton's or Rolfe's framework?

- How easy was it to use?

- What difficulties did you have using it?

- In what ways did it enable you to see the event from a wider perspective?

- How did it enable you to reach alternative conclusions about the event to the ones you had when you started out?

- How has it helped you to frame action that you could take?

- What action did you take?

- How comfortable did you feeling using it?

- Would you choose to use it again?

Try to give the reasons for your answers to these questions.

Of course, what is also seen in using Borton's framework is the beginnings of the reflective spiral. If you take the action that you have identified, it presents you with a continuation of the event, and thus more to reflect on! Many students use this continual spiral to develop deeper and deeper understanding of situations. This is very effective if you are engaged in problem-based learning and need to keep a record of how you gain more knowledge and where it comes from. This can then be used to predict your actions, try them out and reflect further on how your practice has changed as a result of your increased understanding.

KEY POINTS

- Borton's framework leads through the ERA reflective stages completely; hence action is taken as a result of the reflective activity.

- Borton's framework has the simple cue questions of What?, So what? and Now what?

- It is relatively easy to use.

Over to you

The choice of which framework to use for your reflective activity is clearly a choice for you. However, it is worth taking the time to consider why you would select a particular framework, so that you make a conscious decision.

Look back over the critical incidents you have explored using the three models in this chapter.

- Which model did you feel most comfortable using?

- Why was this?

- Would you choose to use this model all the time?

- What are the differences between the models?

- Can you imagine any situations where you would choose to use the different models?

- Would you want to adapt or change them in any ways to suit your particular situations?

CONCLUSIONS

In this chapter you have met three different frameworks for reflection that you can choose to use in your own reflective activities. You will come across others, and may well be given alternatives as part of your own course. The purpose of selecting these three was to provide you with alternatives that have arisen from different disciplines, from different standpoints and for different purposes. All of these are sufficiently flexible to enable you to develop them to suit your own needs. You can, of course, choose to adapt them by adding or leaving out components. You might also find that you create your own framework when you are sufficiently confident at working with the principles of reflection to be able to do so.

If you have been working through the activities in this chapter, you will have created three 'model' cases, each using one of the frameworks that we have presented to you. Each of these will have used a critical incident, so you have also got a clearer understanding of what it means to learn from your own experiences.

Each of these strategies can help us in the quest for developing and changing our practice. Without a doubt, equally useful in achieving this is the act of exploring our own critical incidents. This enables us to build our understanding of our own practice, and to develop our knowledge on the basis of needs that we identify for ourselves.

Finally, the cue to action that arises from engaging in reflective practice is itself a step towards developing our own clinical practice. Each can be used within a variety of reflective situations, and are flexible enough to be used both by yourself and with others.

RAPID RECAP

Check your progress so far by working through each of the following questions.

1 What are Goodman's three levels of reflection?

2 What are the six stages of Gibbs's reflective cycle?

3 What might be a drawback to using Gibbs's cycle within reflective practice?

4 What are the main differences between Gibbs's and Johns' frameworks?

5 What are Carper's types of knowing?

6 What are Borton's three cue questions?

If you have difficulty with more than one of the questions, read through the section again to refresh your understanding before moving on.

REFERENCES

Borton, T. (1970) *Reach, Touch and Teach*. Hutchinson, London.

Carper, B. (1978) Fundamental patterns of knowing in nursing. *Advances in Nursing Science*, **1**, 13–23.

Gibbs, G. (1988) Learning by Doing: A guide to teaching and learning methods. Further Education Unit, Oxford Polytechnic, Oxford.

Goodman, J. (1984) Reflection and teacher education: a case study and theoretical analysis. *Interchanges*, **15**, 9–26.

Health Professions Council (2004) *Standards of conduct, performance and ethics*. Health Professions Council, London. Publication code 034/HPC/A5.

Jacobs-Kramer, M.K. and Chinn, P.L. (1988) Perspectives on knowing: a model of nursing knowledge. *Scholarly Inquiry for Nursing Practice*, **2**, 129–139.

Johns, C. (1998) Opening the doors of perception, in *Transforming Nursing Through Reflective Practice* (eds C. Johns and D. Freshwater), pp. 1–20. Blackwell Science, Oxford.

Johns, C. (2000) *Becoming a Reflective Practitioner*. Blackwell Science, Oxford.

Johns, C. (2006) *Engaging reflection in practice*. Blackwell Scientific Publications, Oxford

Palmer, A., Burns, S. and Bulman, C. (1994) *Reflective Practice in Nursing*. Blackwell Scientific Publications, Oxford.

Rolfe, G., Jasper, M. and Freshwater, D. (2011) *Critical Reflection in Practice: generating knowledge for care*. (2nd edition). Palgrave, Basingstoke.

CHAPTER 4

ENTERING THE WORKING ENVIRONMENT

JOINING YOUR ROLE AS A STUDENT IN THE WORKING ENVIRONMENT

LEARNING OBJECTIVES

By the end of this chapter you should be able to:

- consider your role as a student in the working environment

- anticipate the challenges of entering different working environments

- understand the need to plan your learning experiences in practice to achieve competencies

- consider the role of other people in your learning in practice.

In this chapter you will be thinking about the challenges you may meet when entering the working environment, and how, by anticipating and acknowledging your feelings, worries and anxieties through reflection, you are likely to be more prepared for what you might encounter. The chapter will establish the differing nature of the relationships that you will encounter in the working environment. In particular, it will examine the tensions you will meet in being a student within a workplace, in encountering situations you are not prepared for, which might be unexpected, and in managing unfamiliar situations by drawing on your previous experiences.

Hopefully, this will be a gentle introduction and preparation for going into the working environment and encountering real life situations in practice.

An essential difference between university and your placements is that you will be entering a world whose primary function is to deliver a service to its patients. While you are there to learn, and to learn through observing and providing care under supervision, the others you encounter are there essentially to provide care. Part of their role may be to support learners in the environment, but others you meet will not have a teaching or support component to their job, and although they will recognize you as a student, they are more likely to consider you as simply another worker. This will be especially so of the patients, or clients, that you meet. So, although you know you are a student, many others will not and will have different expectations of you from the ones you have of yourself. It is important, therefore, to think carefully about your role as a student when you go into different working settings, not only to get the most out of the experiences they can offer you but also in terms of:

- the relationships you have with others
- your status within the working environment
- the responsibilities that you have as a student practitioner
- what you need to learn from your placements.

IDENTIFYING YOUR ROLE AS A STUDENT IN THE WORKING ENVIRONMENT

Initially, entering working areas as a student can be very daunting and you will probably experience feelings of anxiety many times as you change placements in order to build up your repertoire of experiences and skills from different settings. No matter what your previous experiences are of working in working environments, when you re-enter as a student your role will be different. You are there primarily to learn. While this learning may occur from actively working in the area or from specific learning opportunities arranged for you, it is your responsibility, working together with your supervisor, to ensure that you achieve the learning that the placement has to offer. In order to maximize your learning from placements it is worth taking some time to think about your role as a student in the working environment, so that you can plan to achieve what you need to from it.

Reflective activity

The nature of learning in university and work placements is very different, as is your role in each one. Try to work through the following questions, either by yourself or with another person, and consider how you can use the different learning environments most effectively to fulfil your learning needs.

1 What are the differences between university and the working arena as learning environments?

2 What opportunities for learning will be available in the working environment?

3 What will the working areas give you that you cannot get from university?

4 What is your role in the working environment?

5 What responsibilities do you have as a student within the working environment in relation to:

- yourself
- the patients and their carers
- the staff with whom you will be working.

6 Who is available to provide you with support in these environments?

7 What else can provide you with guidance while in the working areas?

Above all, the working environments will provide opportunities for developing your knowledge and skills by working with real people in real working settings. As this is the primary purpose of your course, and the ultimate outcome is that you can be licensed to practise as a safe and competent professional, the majority of students find that the working areas are the most enjoyable parts of their study.

However, as working environments, the primary responsibility of most of the other people there is the business of delivering health care. As a result, the role of the student changes from the one in university, where you are the primary focus, to a subsidiary one whose needs come below those of others in the system. Rather than the environment being geared to facilitating your learning, as it is in university, the working areas are designed and organized to provide care to various client groups, and with a range of purposes. Thus the student becomes part of the whole system, not the lynchpin of it.

While your primary reason for being in these environments is to learn from what they have to offer – and this was probably your first answer to question 4 in the previous reflective activity 116 – you will also have a role as a care provider and as a colleague to the other people working in the environment.

For a healthcare student on placement, the working environment is one of many settings.

Your responsibilities to yourself Primarily, it is up to you to ensure that you achieve what you need within your placements. This will include: learning the practical skills of doing the job itself; understanding and developing a professional attitude; remaining safe and reducing the risks you take; and ensuring that your practice falls within the code of professional conduct.

Your responsibilities to your patients These revolve around the notion that you should not cause any harm to anyone in your care. Therefore, not only do you need to be able to deliver effective and high-quality care, you also need to be very clear about the limits of your capabilities and what you are not able to do. You also need to have identified your responsibilities in terms of advocating for others, making decisions for others and being accountable for these under the code of professional conduct and in law. It is very clear that your professional role does not allow you to perform criminal acts towards people in your care. You are liable to both civil and criminal prosecution, as well as disciplinary action from your professional body, if you contravene any of these codes or laws. This includes negligent behaviour or deliberate harm caused to others. Both the Health Care Professions Council and the Nursing and Midwifery Council publish guides for students which you are strongly advised to consult before entering the working environment (HPC 2009, NMC 2011).

Your responsibilities to others in the working environment Even though you are a student, you still have responsibilities to others you are working with. Often these colleagues will have less knowledge than you; or may have habits of working that you, as a person new to the area, can see are not safe. Consider the following case study, written by Carrie, a student nurse on working placement.

Taking the weight

Carrie is a 30-year-old second year adult field nursing student who has previous experience as a health care support worker in an elderly care facility. "Jack, aged 40 years, had been admitted to the ward the previous day having fractured his leg in a road traffic accident. I was working with my mentor when Lisa, a health care support worker, asked me to give her a hand with Jack in the bathroom. He had slipped in the toilet and hurt his other ankle. He was on the floor groaning and said his lower leg hurt. Lisa rushed outside and I assumed she was going for further help. She came back with a wheelchair and asked me to help her to lift Jack into it. Jack was now getting distressed."

tɔɘ11ɘЯ**Reflective activity**

Reflective activity

Decide what you would do next, if you were in the same situation.

Case study

What Carrie decided to do

This is how Carrie reflected on, and learned from, the experience.

"I politely told Lisa that I had been taught not to lift patients manually, (and local guidelines are to always use hoists or other lifting devices where they are available) as there was a great risk of hurting myself, the other lifter and the patient. I made Jack as comfortable as I could, reassured Jack to help calm him down, asked Lisa to stay with him, and went to get the nurse. Lisa said that there was no need as it was only a minor slip, but I told her that we could never be sure so it was safe to let a qualified member of staff know. I then went and explained the situation to my mentor, who came with me to the bathroom to assess Jim and the state of his leg."

tɔɘ11ɘЯ**Reflective activity**

Reflective activity

What were Carrie's responsibilities to Lisa when she was working with her?

If you were in this position, what would be going through your mind in terms of your feelings, and your role as a student?

What, in terms of your knowledge and previous experience, can you use to make sense of this situation?

Case study

Too heavy to handle

Heavy lifting causes accidents in the workplace such as back pain and injury. The Health and Safety Executive (2004) reported over 15000 manual handling accidents in the health care sector and, of these, over 60 per cent were related to patient handling. Forty per cent of sickness absence in the NHS is due to manual handling injuries, costing around £400m (NHS Employers, 2012) Accordingly, all health care organizations must have a Manual Handling policy to benefit both patients and staff. Safe handling often adds up to the quality of care that a patient receives. The Royal College of Nursing (2003) developed a code of practice for handling patients that specified that two nurses should lift no more than 50.8 kg. "I refused to lift Jack because I knew it was wrong according to the Manual Handling policy of the hospital. It was not right for Jack and certainly not right for us as well. I therefore feel that my actions were in everyone's best interests. If we had lifted Jack we might have caused further damage to him, and injured our backs. On reflection, Lisa might have wanted to lift Jack manually because of lack of training, which meant she was unable to identify the risk, or it could just have been to save time as a result of the low staffing levels. Her actions could also have resulted from lack of communication and inadequate information about Jack at handover, which resulted in assumptions about his capabilities.

At the time the incident was happening I felt angry at Lisa, who, after working in the hospital for ten years had failed to adhere to the Manual Handling policy. I also thought she was taking advantage of me as a student, who she thought would agree to do as she was told. When she asked me to lift Jack I felt I had to advocate for him as he had been shocked by the whole event and was unable to speak for himself. My actions were influenced by what I had been taught in class with regard to manual handling and risk assessments. At the back of my mind I could hear the lecturer saying 'Tell them politely that you cannot do it as it is wrong', which I did. I also knew that Jack could not put weight on his right leg because of the plaster cast.

I later had a discussion with my mentor and pointed out that some ward staff had probably done their Manual Handling courses a long time ago and hence needed to be updated with the new policies. She said she would see to it that everyone went on a short course to update their certificates.

I feel, on reflection, that I did the right thing here. I am pleased that none of us were hurt as a result of the incident. Reflecting on this incident has helped me to apply theory to practice, and work according to the code of professional conduct that states that people in the nursing profession should act in such a manner as to safeguard and promote the well-being of patients and others (Nursing and Midwifery Council, 2011). My assertiveness skills were enhanced as I managed to stand my ground by refusing to do what I felt was wrong. I have realized that I can learn from immediate personal experiences in practice. The incident has been a valuable learning experience as I have learned at first hand how to use theories of reflection, and it has encouraged me to think more critically about the ability to use theory in practice. I have also realized that, even though I am a new student, I still have responsibilities to others, even if they are older than me and have more experience.

I do hope that the staff get the updating that they need and that lifting practices change as a result."

References

Health and Safety Executive (2004) *Manual Handling Operations: Guidance on the regulations*, 3nd edn. HSE, London. **http://www.hse.gov.uk/contact/faqs/manualhandling.htm**

National Health Services Employers (2012) *Manual Handling*. **www.nhsemployers.org/Aboutus/Publications/Documents/Manual%20handling.pdf**

Nursing and Midwifery Council (2011) *Guidance on professional conduct for nursing and midwifery students*. NMC, London. **www.nmc-uk.org**

Royal College of Nursing (2003) *Safer staff, better care*. RCN, London.

KEY POINTS

- Remember that you are primarily a student and are placed in practice for the specific purpose of learning from that environment

- Practice placements are working environments – their primary purpose is to deliver care, you will be expected to fit in with the other people there, not the other way round!

- You have responsibilities to the patients and their carers, to other staff and colleagues and to yourself – these are all equally important

- It is normal to experience 'reality shock', anxiety and insecurity when entering new environments; these can be used positively to focus you on what you need to achieve from the experiences available in the placement

Carrie draws attention to the need for assertiveness skills, especially when faced with people attempting to exert their authority over you. Part of your role in working environments will be to act independently and to ensure that you can justify and defend your behaviour and actions at all times. Often this means developing other skills as a student that will carry you forward into self-regulated professional practice. As Carrie has started to be, you will need to be self-empowered as a student to maximize your learning in working placements.

SELF-EMPOWERMENT

So much of what you do during your course is directed by the need to qualify, such as satisfying the professional bodies, completing the specified competencies and achieving the learning outcomes for the course, that it is easy to feel that you have little control yourself.

However, do remember that these outcomes are provided for you as defined endpoints in the course, and the means to achieve them will be offered to you. But it is how you plan to use these, and the attitude you take towards using the experiences on offer within your working placements, that will determine how much you achieve from the breadth of pre-qualifying experiences you have. Taking the opportunities to empower yourself is as much a part of your course as all of the other components.

The reflective cycle provides you with a mechanism for self-empowerment, and the positive reinforcement that you get from being able to take control of your learning will be important to you in feeling that you are part of your own destiny.

Consider Josie's approach to her working placement in the following case study.

Josie has used the ERA reflective cycle effectively here to plan to get the most from her new placement.

Case study

Josie's forward planning

Josie is a third year Occupational Therapy student aged 21 years.

As Josie turned off her light to go to sleep, she was quietly satisfied with her preparations for her new placement, starting the next day. She was looking forward to her placement with the Community Occupational Therapist based in the Social Services Department. Having already completed two years of her course and a range of hospital placements, the next few months were going to be spent in the community experiencing the different working needs and demands of visiting people in their own homes and in residential settings. She even had an alternative placement arranged in America, where she would be visiting a rehabilitation hospital for burns victims.

Josie had taken the time to work out what she needed to achieve from the placement, in terms of both her overall needs for skills required for her job, and the course work she had to complete by the end of the semester. She planned to evaluate and compare the assessment schedules from her last placement with the one used in the community as one assignment. Wanting to focus her dissertation on the specific needs of young, spinally injured patients retraining for new careers, she had liaised with her new supervisor to spend time with the Occupational Therapist in the local residential unit.

She was confident that she would get on well with Jane, her community supervisor, as she had spoken to her on the phone already and they had talked about the competencies that she needed to achieve from this placement. As a result, she knew that Jane had planned a schedule of visits, both by herself and with other members of staff, to give her the experiences that she needed. She had also mentioned her assignments and assessment schedule, so that Jane would be aware of what she was doing in her study time and could look out for anything happening that would help with those. Finally, Josie had worked out a rough time plan for getting the work completed this semester so that she wouldn't feel under too much pressure. Her bag was packed for tomorrow and she had made sure that she had her competencies and assessment documents with her so that she and Jane could really put their first morning together to good use. Time was going so fast now, with finals looming, and she felt that she couldn't afford to miss any opportunities to get closer to fulfilling the packed schedule of the last nine months of the course. As she went to sleep that night she was confident that she had done all that she could to get the most out of this placement.

The *event* itself was to be the upcoming placement in the community. The stages of the reflective cycle can be broken down and applied in the following way.

Stage 1: Identifying the experience/critical incident Josie started from the point of identifying what it was that she needed to achieve by looking at her assessment schedule, her competency document and the opportunities that would be available in the community. She was also anticipating her needs following that in terms of her elective placement and her dissertation.

Stage 2: Observing and describing the experience From these Josie was able to anticipate what it was she wanted to achieve from the working placement. These she had phrased as learning needs that matched her outcomes. She was able to predict what opportunities would be available in her new placement.

Stage 3: Analyzing the experience Josie was then able to break down the opportunities available, on the basis of her previous knowledge and experience and what she had been told by her lecturers, her new supervisor and her student colleagues, and match these to her learning needs.

Stage 4: Interpreting the experience From the experience available within the working placement she was able to select what was appropriate and most likely to enable her to achieve what she wanted. She also realized that there were unknowns that would be encountered, and that these would add to the breadth of her experiences.

Stage 5: Exploring alternatives Having realized that there were competencies that she needed to develop but were not already planned by her supervisor, she explored other ways of getting these. This included asking Jane if she could spend extended time at the spinal injuries intermediate care unit to gather information for her dissertation. She also wanted to apportion her time so that she could complete the comparative assignment on OT assessment from the examples she found in the community. All of these meant that she was making the most of the opportunities that might be available, and gearing them specifically to her own learning needs.

Stage 6: Framing action Josie planned to phone Jane to ensure that her perceptions and ideas were on the right lines. She was also anxious about the first meeting with Jane and wanted to know what she sounded like to allay her fears. She planned an assessment schedule to complete her assignments for this semester on time in order to take the pressure off and know that she was planning to complete her work by the submission dates. She provisionally ticked off the competencies for this placement, and also those that came from other sections, in her book so she knew she hadn't overlooked anything.

Finally, Josie completed the ERA cycle by carrying out the action that she had planned. She had spoken to Jane and ensured that she knew when and where she was expected the following day. She had packed her bag and ensured that she had the documents with her that she needed. Her time plan and work schedule were on her wall. She knew what she hoped to achieve during the placement, and was content that there was not much more she could have done in preparation.

Josie might appear to be the 'model' student, yet all that she had done was to choose to spend a couple of hours in reflection and forward planning. As a result she did achieve her required competencies, her assignments and the extra things that she had wanted to get from the experience. Her deliberate use of time in reflection in this way actually saved her time overall, as she wasn't wasting her energy worrying about not having enough time or having to catch up with things that could have been planned in advance.

Contrast this with Justin's approach, in the following case study.

Case study

Justin lives for the moment

'So, what is it that you need to achieve from your placement in Intensive Care then, Justin?' asked Kerrie.

'Er... well, I haven't really thought about it. Until I see what you do and what goes on here, I won't know, will I?' replied Justin.

'OK, so let's think about your assignments then, and your competencies for this semester. What university work do you have to do that we can tie in with your placement here?' said Kerrie, hoping that this might provide a focus for what was turning out to be a difficult first meeting with her student.

'I don't know. I think we may have an ethics assignment, and I suppose I need to start thinking about a dissertation topic. But to be quite honest, I don't have a clue', replied Justin.

'Well, think about that and we'll talk about it later in the week. Now, your competencies – let's see what else you have left to cover and what we need to plan to include in your time here'.

'Um… well, I haven't got it with me, I forgot it in the rush to get out this morning. Had a late night with the boys last night and didn't get much sleep. You know how it goes….'

In fact, Justin is a classic case of a student who thinks that life simply happens – and that his failure to get work in on time, get good marks, achieve his competencies and find his course interesting has nothing to do with him. As a result, he considered himself to be disorganized and a failure, and envied others who appeared to sail through life with no problems. He had a record of late submissions, not knowing where he was going, turning up to placements late and misunderstanding what work needed to be done. Consequently, despite being a likeable and personable student, his tutors and working assessors doubted that he had the attitude or strength of character to act responsibly and independently as a professional practitioner. He lacked neither academic nor working ability, but he was totally oblivious to the fact that all these things were under his control.

He couldn't see that, in failing to assess and plan his course, he was not developing the independence and organizational capacities that would be expected of him when qualified and responsible and accountable for his own actions, and those of others.

Over to you

Take some time to think about your usual approach to starting a new placement. Are you a Josie or a Justin?

While these students represent the two extremes of behaviour, it is likely that you recognize some of these characteristics in yourself. For instance:

- Do you forward plan when going into new situations?
- Do you identify your goals and what you want to achieve?
- Do you set yourself time schedules?
- Do you blame other people for things that go wrong in your life?
- Do you see things as beyond your control – such as not having enough time to do things?
- Do you feel sometimes that you are lacking in ability, and that this is why you don't get good marks, or fail exams?

What can you learn from your answers to these questions?

Do you need to change your behaviour in any way so that you can plan to achieve what you want to, rather than less, as you often do through failing to plan?

This section has been about empowering yourself as a student. Empowerment is about taking responsibility for our own actions. Empowerment as a student is about enabling yourself to achieve what you need for the future. To be empowered, we need sufficient information to make decisions and the drive to plan on the basis of that information. Perhaps more importantly, though, is that we need to believe in ourselves, in our own capacity and ability to achieve what we want to. An attitude needs to be adopted that says 'I can and I will'. One way to do this is to plan for the future and be determined to carry out those plans. Who do you think will be successful in their lives – Josie or Justin? Can you identify your reasons for thinking this?

IDENTIFYING LEARNING EXPERIENCES IN THE WORKING ENVIRONMENT

Within reflective practice the experiences you have are used as the foundations for actively, and consciously, learning in a professional capacity. Throughout your professional education, and in all of the placements you gain practical experience, you will build up a range of different situations and examples that provide the foundations of your professional knowledge. While it is impossible to reflect actively on all these, it is the conscious reflection on some of them that will enable you to capitalize on what you are doing and recognize that you are learning as you progress through your course. In a way, reflective practice is a short cut to learning. You will learn more quickly if you get into the habit of reflecting on your experiences, identifying the learning that you have achieved and the action that you need to take as a result.

Reflective activity

Why do you do what you do?

It is worth taking the time to think about the different opportunities and sources of experience that may arise from the working environment. Take a few minutes to reflect on the nature of the working environment. Identify the types of experience and situation you may encounter that will provide opportunities for learning.

For instance:

- What ways do you use to learn in the university setting?
- How will learning in the working environment differ from learning in a university setting?
- What things can you do to ensure that you learn in these environments?
- What can you do to ensure that you recognize your learning?

- How can you draw on other people to help you learn in working environments?
- What responsibilities do you have for organizing your learning in the working environment?
- What is available to help and guide you in identifying and organizing these responsibilities?

There are different ways that we can think about these opportunities, and many of these will have been included in your list.

LEARNING FROM OTHERS

As a student you will always be working under the supervision of a qualified member of staff, and will meet other professionals in the course of your experiences. You will also meet many other people in different professions, as clients and carers, as users of health care services and as colleagues and co-workers in support services. These people each offer different opportunities for learning.

Your supervisor

Initially, it is primarily from your supervisor that you will be learning, as you use him/her as a role model for the way that you act in the working environment. Together you will work on identifying what it is you need to learn and on planning your experiences so that you have the opportunities to achieve these goals. The relationship between yourself and your supervisor is a relatively formal one, as it may be the supervisor who assesses your progress and competence. The supervisor is ultimately responsible for you while you are in the workplace and is accountable for the actions that you undertake under their professional supervision. They need to ascertain your capabilities for themselves before trusting you to take responsibility with patients. Therefore, it is here that you are likely to be able to gain structure in planning your experiences in the working environment, and work towards meeting planned goals and objectives through your supervisor's guidance and support. Your supervisor will be your first contact in the placement and the initial person you will turn to throughout the time you spend in the area. Your supervisor is also likely to be the lynchpin around which the whole placement revolves, as they know the area, the types of opportunities available and the specific strengths and skills of other members of staff.

Other qualified staff and students in your own professional field

You will, of course, work with many others in your own working speciality. This might happen in a formal or informal way. For instance, another practitioner may have been asked to work with you for the day because they have particular expertise or are going to visit a certain client who offers you experience of certain conditions that you might not get with your supervisor. This is particularly the case where practitioners hold their own caseloads and have built up experience over many years in one area of practice. Your supervisor may decide that others can offer you a wider range of experiences in this way than they can themselves. In addition, you will have many opportunities for discussion with your own colleagues.

Working with others in your own chosen profession, whether they are your supervisors or other qualified staff, enables you to learn, and take on, the attributes of being a practitioner in this particular profession – these are called socialization processes.

These socialization processes enable you to function within your own professional world. They include becoming familiar with the language, ways of working, attitudes, skills and professional attributes that go along with your profession. It is almost impossible to acquire these without working with others. It is similar to learning the rules of a game in order to win. You learn these by observing and mimicking the ways in which your role models conduct themselves as practitioners. In this way, you will build up the attributes that make you acceptable to others in your profession; and other attributes will become extinct. You may find that you admire and respect some people more than others and deliberately try to adopt the ways in which they work. Other people may not impress you so much and you may catch yourself making a mental note not to emulate their behaviour. Use your experiences of working with others in your field as a focus for reflection. This will enable you to work on becoming the type of practitioner who exhibits these features, so that you become recognizable as a member of that profession. You will also find that you become more comfortable with others as a result, as you start to display those attributes yourself and fit in with the others around you.

Over to you

Look back to the reflective activity on professional attributes in Chapter 2 (page 42).

Your answers to the last three questions in this activity will have begun to clarify for you the type of image that you admire in a practitioner. They will have started to set standards for you to achieve as you develop and acquire an identity as one of those practitioners yourself. In learning about professional practice, we tend to unconsciously emulate those around us with whom we can identify. In doing this exercise, you will now be more aware of the characteristics and attributes of others that you can consciously make a note of and consider in light of your own development and behaviour. An example of how this happened to one student nurse is described in the following case study.

Case study

Witnessing unprofessional behaviour

Martha is a 30-year-old 2nd year Adult field nursing student. She is also a single mother, living with her four-year-old daughter near to her own parents within the Afro-Caribbean community. The incident took place in the ward office during handover. A 15-year-old girl, Anne, had been admitted to the ward two days before to have a lump removed from her left leg. She was also six months pregnant. Her mum, Mrs West, had been very worried about her and was constantly by her side during visiting times. The day Anne had her operation she was in a lot of pain and her mum wanted to stay with her all night. The night staff did not permit her to do so as it was against hospital regulations. Mrs West was,

however, assured that her daughter would be well cared for and that she would be contacted if the need arose. She did not like the arrangement and became abusive, but left eventually and returned early the next morning.

During handover, Sister Stringer said:

'Oh, that Mrs West and her daughter are trouble makers! The mum didn't want to leave last night and made so much noise about it. Anyway, it's not as if her daughter is the first to have an operation, and it's certainly not our fault that she is pregnant at 15. Watch out for them'.

She then went on to say that Anne needed a 'motherectomy' because of the attitude and behaviour of her mother. Sister was saying all this without realizing that the door was not fully closed and that Mrs West happened to be passing by just then. Mrs West heard everything that was said.

Everyone in the office froze with fright and embarrassment. It was agreed that Sister should apologize but she refused to do so as she felt she had told the truth.

Reflective activity

What are your initial reactions to this incident?

How would you have felt if you had been a witness?

What are your impressions about the behaviour of the ward sister in:

- Saying what she said in handover in the first place?
- Refusing to apologize to the patient?

Case study

Martha continued her account

"I felt so offended and disgusted about the whole incident. I could not understand how Sister could

speak about human beings, people for whom we were meant to be caring, in this way. While Sister may have tried some irreverent humour, which many nurses do in isolation because of the pressures of the job, by saying 'motherectomy', this went beyond humour. I would have found this surprising in itself, coming from someone with her status and authority, but to have it witnessed by the person she was referring to was just awful. The whole episode was a culture shock for me, especially as it was said during a handover, which is meant to be a factual presentation of the patients between shifts. A handover is a powerful medium, as information shared at that time stays with us for the rest of the shift. If someone is described in a certain way, it can sometimes be difficult to step aside from that description and really assess a person on their own qualities; thus patients become labelled, and it is difficult as the practitioner to put that aside once it has been heard. I really felt that what Sister had said was very unfair because she was forming an opinion for all of us based on her feelings."

While Sister may have felt that she had only said what had happened, her manner was not professional at all. It is important as health professionals to always show cultural sensitivity, respect equality and be open-minded. Although it was right for Sister to relay information to us, it was not right for her to be judgemental and express her personal opinions. The manner in which information and confidences are shared is a sensitive indicator of whether professional attitudes are creating dependency or whether they are used to assist patients towards autonomy and help them take control of their own lives. This means that, if the handover information had been said as if Anne and her mother were present, no one would have been hurt, the Sister would not have looked unprofessional and the rest of the staff would not have been so embarrassed. Sister's actions show that she was not acting in the best interests of the patient and her carers. As professionals, treating people as unique individuals involves respecting their rights at all times (NMC, 2011). In this case, the fact that Anne was pregnant should not have been an issue for Sister, it was nothing to do with the reason that she had been admitted. While Mrs West might have been a nuisance to the ward staff, her behaviour was out of concern for her daughter – being treated with care and consideration by the nursing staff would have helped to allay her anxieties and made the experience a more positive one for both of them. By showing such negative feelings towards Anne and her mother, Sister showed a lack of pastoral care and empathy.

The impression that Anne and her mother have of nurses is that they gossip and are untrustworthy. If Sister had apologized for what she had said, this might have been rectified. But she compounded the problem by refusing to say sorry for what she had said.

Reflective activity

What have you learned from this case study about the responsibilities that we have as professionals when referring to patients? How do you feel about the ward sister's refusal to apologize?

What are the differences between the ways in which we refer to others when we are acting in a professional capacity and the sorts of thing we can say in private?

Are there any implications arising from your code of professional conduct that you might refer to here?

What impressions might the public gain, from incidents like this, about the ways in which professionals act?

In terms of your own future behaviour, what decisions can you take now about the ways in which you will talk about your patients to other people when acting in a professional capacity?

This is how Martha summarized her learning

"I have learned that privacy is of the utmost importance during handovers in order to protect information shared during that time. Personal feelings should not interfere with handovers, and we should not give our opinions about other people, whether we approve of their behaviour or not. We should instead concentrate on factual information and patients' needs for care. I hope I would apologize if I offended a patient in any way.

I have also learned that there are boundaries between our role as a professional and our role as a private person. In nursing, because we are with patients for extended periods of time, it is easy to slip into being friendly and maybe muddying the differences between how we would act as a professional and how we would act as a friend. It is important for me to develop professional ways of relating to people, and I have learned here that it is very easy to cross those boundaries. I will be careful to keep my personal views about people to myself, or perhaps to only share them when I am away from the working area, where I can give my viewpoints, rather than being in a professional working relationship.

I now also appreciate how important recognizing good role models will be for my development. This incident was a crucial one for me as it was so extreme. I had heard other nurses hand over before and say things like 'He's a lovely gentleman' or 'He's a dirty old man' and really thought nothing of it. But this incident has really brought it home to me how inappropriate it is to make personal remarks about anyone. I think the rule of never saying anything about anyone that you wouldn't say in front of them is a really good one, and one that I will try to always observe in the future.

I have gained much from reflecting on this incident. The structured process has intensified my self-awareness and made me analyze the extent to which my own thoughts, feelings and actions can affect the provision of quality nursing care. Reflection has been a good learning experience for me and is certainly a tool I will use throughout my practice to identify areas of practice that I think are in need of further development, and those areas that may already have been successfully developed."

QUALIFIED STAFF AND STUDENTS IN OTHER PROFESSIONAL FIELDS

Similarly, in today's multidisciplinary health care world, you will always be encountering practitioners and students from other professions. These people will provide you with differing perspectives on caring for others from those that come from your own profession.

**Working with many different health care professions
enriches your professional development.**

Over to you

Take some time now to think about the features of some of the different health care professions that you have met.

First, write down the features of your own profession. For instance, think about:

- What it was that attracted you to this profession instead of others
- The key features of your profession, i.e. what distinguishes you from other health care workers
- What type of care you provide to patients
- The environment in which you provide that care
- The nature of the relationship you have with patients
- The type of education that prepares practitioners
- The relationships you have with other professional groups
- The degree of independence your profession has within the health care field

Now, using the same identifying features, compare these with at least two other professional groups. Those you might choose from are:

- Nurses
- Midwives
- Physiotherapists

- Occupational therapists
- Radiographers
- Social workers
- Operating department practitioners
- Paramedics
- Speech and language therapists
- Doctors
- Working psychologists
- Dietitians

Finally, think about what you could learn from these other groups that will help your own development as a practitioner. How can these groups complement the care that you provide for patients? If you had the opportunity to spend time with people from these professions, what is it that you would want to gain from that experience?

Making the most of other people's experience is important for you in developing your own skills. Very few practitioners work in isolation in caring for patients. You will increasingly find yourself attending team meetings and discussions involving a range of workers from different disciplines, all of whom provide their own perspective on caring for the patient they are focussing on. It is by understanding the parameters within which these professionals work, and the areas of expertise and responsibility they have, that you will come to develop a deeper understanding of your own role. But you will also learn to appreciate the alternative skills and perspectives that others bring to problems and situations, which will broaden your understanding of working within a multidisciplinary workforce.

KEY POINTS

- Identify the other people in each placement that can help you to achieve your learning needs
- Develop a working relationship with your supervisor that focuses on what you need to get from the placement
- Remember that your supervisor is also likely to be your assessor and is a practitioner in their own right, with roles and responsibilities defined by codes of professional conduct and the supervisor's contract of employment
- Other qualified practitioners in your own field, and from other disciplines, have a wealth of experience that they are willing to share – try to capitalize on this when planning your learning and experiences
- Remember that we have responsibilities to our patients, co-workers and other students – we may have more information and knowledge than they do

While learning from working with other people is very important, you will also find you can learn from what is going on around you, in terms of the opportunities available in the specific working context of your placement.

LEARNING FROM WORKING PLACEMENTS

During your course your working placements will be selected to ensure that you have the opportunities to experience a broad range of health care settings and contexts. Each one offers different experiences for you to develop knowledge, skills and competencies contributing to your overall development as a practitioner. Over the length of your course, it is likely that you will only visit each specialty once, and therefore it is very important that you plan to gain as much from the placement as it has to offer.

At other times you may experience client attachment or caseload allocation. These offer a different sort of experience, where you learn through building up your experiences by assessing, planning and providing care. These types of placements offer the experience of relatively long-term interactions with patients, where you follow a person through their encounter with your particular service, and therefore you build up your own bank of paradigm cases from which to draw on later in your professional life.

Your placements will be divided into mainstream placements and alternative placements. Mainstream placements will help you to build the essential characteristics of your own profession, and achieve the competencies and standards required for qualification. Alternative placements offer extra experiences during which you also learn your role. These may be dependent on your own interests within a particular field and on the types of opportunity available. Many courses offer optional or elective placements where students are able to choose where they go; some may even be in a different country or health care system, in a different part of the country or specialty, or in specialist working areas that develop skills not normally expected in pre-qualifying experience.

Paradigm cases
Separate cases that we build up as a repertoire of experience and use to reflect back to when we meet similar experiences again

Reflective activity

Take some time now to think about the types of experience offered during your course. Even if you only know your placements for a few months, or this year, you can still reflect on the learning that you will be able to achieve from them.

- How many of these placements are designed to provide you with the core knowledge, skills and experience that characterize your profession?

- What are these placements?

- How will these contribute to the way you meet the competencies and standards for your professional registration?

- What other placements will you be experiencing?

- How will these supplement your learning from your core placements?

Of course, the many professional groups involved in health care delivery mean that each professional group has a different way of organizing care, and therefore can offer different types of experience. For instance, operating department practitioners (ODPs) have very specific roles in working with patients who are undergoing surgical procedures. However, this activity may not be confined to operating theatres alone. Anywhere that an anaesthetic could be administered and patients need to be cared for while under its influence would offer experience for students. So, outpatient clinics where patients undergo minor procedures, or X-ray departments where investigations are done, may also be offering working placements for student ODPs. Similarly, the student ODP needs to know what happens to patients before they get to the operating department, in terms of preparation for their operation. This is particularly important where complicated surgery will be taking place, or where surgery may have long term consequences. So a student ODP may also be offered short-term placements in an intensive care unit or on a general surgical ward in order to develop their perspective of their own specialty. This enables the student to place their care within the context of care delivered by the other professional disciplines. The following case study shows how one ODP student broadened his perspective of caring for patients while in an observational placement.

Case study

Seeing the whole person

Kemi is a 35-year-old ODP student just entering the second and final year of her programme. She is working in a ward to gain alternative experience, and in particular develop her communication skills with patients undergoing procedures under local anaesthetic.

"During the night Mrs Jones, a 78-year-old lady, was admitted to the ward with a fractured left wrist following a fall. She also had multi-infarct dementia and lived in a nursing home. She was classified as nil-by-mouth on arrival in anticipation of corrective surgery. At 14.30 a nurse and I took Mrs Jones to the trauma room in A&E as the fractured wrist was to be treated conservatively (without surgery). The doctor was to manipulate the bone back into the correct position, thus reducing the fracture, after

which the wrist would be immobilized in a back slab plaster. The procedure was to be done under a general anaesthetic and so the doctor hadn't administered morphine before moving her from the ward as it wouldn't be necessary and, as a respiratory depressant, would be a risk for Mrs Jones. When we arrived, however, he said that he would use a local anaesthetic after all. The nurse suggested that Mrs Jones was given morphine and that the procedure was delayed until it took effect. Attempts to explain what was happening to Mrs Jones were unsuccessful because of her dementia and she became very agitated. As a result she flailed as the doctor was injecting the local anaesthetic, causing her arm to bleed. Despite the anaesthetic and analgesic, it was clear that Mrs Jones was in a considerable amount of pain when her wrist was manipulated. She wriggled a lot and started shouting. At this point the doctor, who was holding Mrs Jones' left hand, asked me to hold her left arm above the elbow to keep her still enough for the cast to be applied.

This incident provoked a number of feelings in me. Firstly, I was confused about the lack of communication regarding the procedure – the nursing team had been under the impression that a general anaesthetic was to be used. During the procedure I felt useless; there was little I could do to assist apart from helping to hold Mrs Jones still and attempting to reassure and distract her. Most of all I felt guilty because as a team we were causing the patient so much pain. I felt worse knowing that it wasn't just the orthopaedic procedure that was causing her pain but also our attempts to keep her still. I also felt slightly angry because, as a student ODP on observation, I did not feel able to question the events in any way.

On the positive side, Mrs Jones was asleep half an hour after the procedure, remembered nothing of the event and returned to her nursing home the next day. I gained empirical knowledge, observed an orthopaedic procedure done under local that I would not have seen otherwise and learned a little about the realities of dealing with patients with dementia. Usually when these patients come to theatre they are heavily sedated and we don't have to cope with their behaviour, even in the recovery room. On the negative side, the incident could have been handled a lot better. Firstly, the lack of communication resulted in Mrs Jones being nil-by-mouth for 13 hours. Not only was this unnecessary and must have caused discomfort, it could also result in dehydration, which interferes with normal bodily processes. Where a patient is unable to communicate effectively with the caring staff this is even more dangerous and could have serious consequences. Secondly, it resulted in inadequate sedation and analgesia, causing Mrs Jones more pain and distress than she should have had.

I have learned a great deal from this incident in terms of the need to treat patients individually. This often gets overlooked in theatres as patients are listed for procedures and we rarely interact with them as people. Reducing this fracture under general anaesthetic would have been an easier and more straightforward procedure but was not the most appropriate course of action for Mrs Jones because of her age and anaesthetic risk. My role under these circumstances was different from my normal one, and yet it is becoming more likely given the expanding role of ODPs into different working situations. I have realized that I take comfort from the fact that patients are usually unconscious and that I don't have to offer emotional support or think about not causing them pain. I appreciate now the role that nurses often play in reassuring and supporting patients in order to reduce anxiety and gain co-operation, and that these are skills that I will need to learn. This placement has been a very valuable learning experience in that I now see people more as individuals with different needs than simply as procedures on a list."

All working placements will offer you alternative experiences and will have been chosen, and audited, for their potential educational value in contributing to your experience. Sometimes you may be disappointed that you have not got the placement that you wanted, but making the most of what any placement offers is an important skill to develop, despite your feelings about it. Planning to use the placement for what it can offer you and how it can help you to achieve your learning outcomes is a positive way of approaching new placements. This can be done by analyzing the context of the placement and anticipating the types of opportunities and experiences that it can offer. The following checklist will help you in doing this.

Check list to use in evaluating the potential of a working placement

- What is the specialty of the placement?
- What are the characteristics of the patients it deals with in terms of:

  – age
  – sex
  – reason for being a patient and/or
  – reason for being under the care of your professional group
  – other specific criteria, e.g. immobility, disability?

- What is the range of experience that it can offer you?
- What specific experiences and/or events are available here?
- What skills/competencies will you achieve here?
- How will this placement contribute to your attainment of the standards for practice?
- How will this placement contribute to your overall course outcomes?

Much of your learning in placements will come from specific events, such as critical incidents, that happen to you.

KEY POINTS

- Placements are unique and offer unique experiences
- Analyze your placements to identify what they can offer against your learning needs
- Plan to use your placements to achieve your objectives

LEARNING FROM EVENTS

Clearly, whenever you are in placements in the working environment, things will be going on around you all the time. In fact, so much will be happening that you will find it impossible to take everything in that occurs while you are there! There are two ways that we can look at this.

Firstly, we can allow things to wash over us and just experience them as they happen. This is what we will do most of the time, and we will slowly absorb the ways of working and doing things as we become familiar with what is going on.

Secondly, however, we may consciously decide to focus on events that are happening and make them a feature of our reflective practice. In these instances we will be selecting from everything that is happening for a particular purpose.

In the second case, the reasons we decide to concentrate on a particular event are important. Some of these reasons may be:

- It is selected for you by your supervisor because it is something that they feel you need to do at that time
- Because you need to experience and learn one thing before you are able to go on and do others
- Because that event happens irregularly and therefore you need to make the most of when it does occur
- Because different skills or ways of doing something will be on offer that your supervisor feels will broaden your experience
- Because you have specific learning outcomes for that placement
- Because this experience is only likely to be available from this placement.

Making the most of events that are occurring is important in enabling you to get the most from what is on offer. Many experiences cannot be predicted; others can. It is up to you, along with your supervisor, to ensure that you select from what is available in any placement to ensure that you gain the experiences that you need as a practitioner. One of the ways in which you may identify these is through your course competencies and the outcomes expected for professional registration.

KEY POINTS

- Analyze each placement for the specific events that occur that you need or want to experience
- Arrange your placement time/shifts so that you are there when they happen
- Tell your supervisor, or the other people that you are working with, if there is anything that you want to be able to experience whilst on that placement

LEARNING FROM COURSE STRUCTURE, COMPETENCIES, PROFESSIONAL BODY STANDARDS AND COURSE OUTCOMES

Your course will be organized and structured in a way to ensure that you experience and achieve what you need in order to qualify in your chosen profession. How this is structured derives from the experience of your lecturers and supervisors in practice. Similarly, the placements that are organized for you will have been selected with specific objectives in mind. After all, you cannot learn everything at once! Each unit, or module of study, will have specified learning outcomes. Similarly, your stage in the course provides expectations about your knowledge, skills and what you can do in the practical environment. You will be expected to build on foundation skills and knowledge as you progress through the course, incrementally developing your way to competence as a practitioner in your own right.

Using outcomes and professional body standards for practice to structure your learning experiences is a useful way of ensuring that you achieve everything that you need. By identifying what it is that you need to achieve, you can assess what is on offer in a particular placement and plan to achieve the outcomes, or competencies, which will be available there. This does take active planning and review at specific points during the placement to assess whether you are on track. Both your work supervisor and academic tutor will be available to help you.

With all of these having been given to you, your main job is to make the most of the opportunities that are presented in the working environment. This will ensure that you learn from the broadest possible range of experiences available in your protected time as a pre-qualifying student. This will happen if you spend some of your private study time planning what it is you need to achieve, and how you will do this during the different stages of your course.

Over to you

Construct a checklist for evaluating specific events that you may come across in your placements. Use the one in the previous section to provide cue questions that you can use when selecting and reflecting on events that may be available as experiences in placements. Try to relate these to your course or module outcomes; to assignments that you may need to complete; or to working or practical competencies.

It may be that you can use one event for several different purposes. For instance, reflecting on one critical incident may enable you to provide evidence of having achieved a couple of competencies, and satisfy a written course work assignment demonstrating your ability to use a reflective framework. This whole piece of work may then be included in your portfolio as evidence of your ongoing development and gradual achievement of the course outcomes. Using the same event for different outcomes also enables you to see the links between theory and practice, and the integration of the different components of the course. Reflective processes and practice are not strategies that can be separated out from the reality of being a practitioner. They cannot occur in the abstract because they depend on real life for their subject matter. So, although you are being encouraged to focus specifically on them while a student, they are like any other skill or technique that you use in your professional development in that they do not stand alone but, rather, are incorporated into everything you do.

KEY POINTS

- Use the information that you have been given about your course structure, assignments and competencies to plan to get the most out of your working placements

- Spend time at the beginning of the placement in planning what you will be able to achieve from what you need to achieve

SELF-DIRECTED LEARNING AND INDIVIDUAL INTERESTS

Finally, your own interests and needs will help to provide some direction in selecting what you choose to use as active learning experiences. These might arise from your evaluation of what your strengths and weaknesses are, of what your own professional interests are or of the type of specialty that you want to go into when you qualify. The time you spend on your course will provide you with a range of opportunities that you are unlikely to encounter in such a short space of time again in your career. While the purpose of your course is to enable you to develop an acceptable level of competence as a practitioner so that you can safely be allowed to be responsible for patient care, your registration as a practitioner is simply the beginning of another stage in your learning.

After qualification you will begin to build your skills, knowledge and expertise directed by your own interests and aptitudes, as opposed to those directed for you by the needs of registration and regulation. This flexibility brings with it another set of responsibilities as you become your own guide for your professional learning needs. This process starts, like all others, during the pre-qualifying period, in that there will always be self-identified and self-directed learning needs that arise over and above those specified in your course. It is likely that many of these will arise from the experiences that you have in working placements. As you find that you want to know more about what you are encountering, you will realize that the generic knowledge learned in university is insufficient for the specific experiences that occur in the real world of patient care. Thus, much of your reflective learning from placements will arise from the unique experiences you have throughout your course. Using these as a focus for reflective practice will therefore broaden your base for professional practice.

Your self-directed and independent learning, just like all the other opportunities that you have, will need to be focused in particular ways. As a student, this is usually done by screening out things that are not essential to success in your course. Hence, when selecting what to spend your self-directed time on, you will need to ask yourself specific, needs-related questions and be instrumental in how you use your time. You will find that you can 'double-count' much of what you are doing by ensuring that you use many, if not all, of what you do for at least two purposes. Many of these incidences will arise by combining the requirements of your course with your own interests. You might, for instance:

- Choose to focus an assignment on a subject matter that is of specific interest to you
- Select a critical incident that enables you to explore your own interests while achieving several competencies or learning outcomes in the course
- Ensure that the topic of your final project or dissertation is related to the specialty of the placement/s you will be in at the time
- Select elective placements, particularly towards the end of your course, that enable you to develop skills and contacts for employment on qualification.

Over to you

We all have criteria that help us decide how we will use our time. Try to develop a list of your own that will guide your self-directed study and that reflects your needs as a student in planning to complete your course successfully. The following questions may help you to do this, but you will probably want to add more of your own.

- Why have I chosen to read/study/write about this topic?
- How does it fit with the stage/requirements of the course at this moment?
- How will it help me to achieve this semester's/year's academic assignments?
- How will it inform my practical placements?
- How will it contribute to my knowledge for my future practice?
- Does it contribute to the competencies I need to demonstrate?
- What am I trying to achieve in doing it?
- Do I have the time to do it?
- Do I really need to do it?
- Do I really want to do it?

As you progress through your course, you will find that you are drawn to some elements of practice more than others and that these are where you choose to specialize when you qualify. The nature of most professional practice in contemporary health care means that practitioners choose specialist areas of practice very soon after qualification. For many of you this will not be a conscious decision. This may be because you have a broad range of interests and do not have any particular leanings towards one or another. Others know at an early stage in their course just where their interests lie and choose to specialize swiftly after initial qualification by going on to further courses or working in designated areas of their practice. These areas of interest are often founded in our pre-qualifying experiences.

KEY POINTS

- We learn best where our interest is stimulated – so try to focus as much of your required course components as you can through your own specific interests

- We tend to be 'needs' motivated as students – in other words, we focus our time on what we need to do, rather than what we want to do. If we can find ways of combining these, and double counting our experiences in working environments, we are more likely to achieve our goals successfully

- Your pre-qualifying course is simply a preparation for the rest of your professional life – so try to use your working experiences constructively for the future. Look out for opportunities that will establish the foundations for your career as a practitioner

CONCLUSIONS

The learning achieved from your working experiences and placements is the link between theory and practice. As practitioners we can only make sense of theory if we apply it, see it in action, reflect on it and discover our own knowledge base derived from this unique combination. Every practitioner has a different knowledge base for practice arising from the experiences they have had – no two practitioners have ever had the same experiential basis for their learning. Hence, no two practitioners can be said to have the same knowledge base. As practitioners, our skill lies in safe and competent practice, in being able to select from alternatives and predict outcomes for our patients. We need to have confidence in and justify our professional decisions and actions. We need to acknowledge the limitations of our own practice and be prepared to listen to others, or invite them in to share the care of our patients. None of this can be learned from theory alone.

As a student you have the privilege of being able to study in the real world. Within this world there is a wealth of opportunities available for learning your craft. These opportunities range from the people you meet, to the specialist services encountered, the events and experiences that happen opportunistically or as planned occurrences, and our natural tendencies in terms of interests and motivation.

The key to getting the most out of working placements and environments is in planning your experiences to ensure that you identify the opportunities they offer and maximizing how they help you to achieve your outcomes. Reflective processes and practice provide the strategies for you to do this, whether these are used in anticipation of your working experiences or retrospectively after events have occurred.

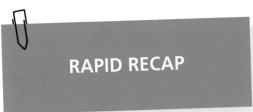

RAPID RECAP

Check your progress so far by working through each of the following questions.

1   What is the primary difference between the university environment and the practice environment?

2   To whom do you have responsibilities in the working environment?

3   What are your roles as a student in the practice environment?

4   What is meant by 'self-empowerment'?

5   What are the different types of learning opportunities available in working practice?

6   What is meant by the term 'socialization processes'?

7   How can we get the most out of the opportunities available for learning in practice?

If you have difficulty with more than one of the questions, read through the section again to refresh your understanding before moving on.

REFERENCES

Health Professions Council (2009) *Guidance on conduct and ethics for students*. 3rd edition. HPC, London.

Nursing and Midwifery Council (2011) *Guidance on professional conduct for nursing and midwifery students*. NMC, London.

CHAPTER 5

WAYS OF REFLECTING ON YOUR OWN

LEARNING OBJECTIVES

By the end of this chapter you should be able to:

- identify ways of reflecting that suit your learning style

- explore a range of reflective strategies that can be used for personal reflection

- identify the differences between written reflective strategies and other ways of reflecting

- consider the ways in which you can use reflective writing within your portfolio.

While the previous chapters have worked at setting up the foundations for and ideas behind reflective practice, these next two present practical ways to enable you to be a reflective practitioner.

The aim of this chapter is to introduce you to a variety of strategies for reflecting by yourself. We start by revisiting the idea of actively working with your learning style, before moving on to the two principal ways in which you will reflect by yourself – thinking things over and writing reflectively. While both these approaches share common elements, they each have individual features that contribute separately to the techniques you will use to learn and understand about practice. Some use the frameworks for reflection introduced in Chapter 3; others are more creative and therefore provide a range of approaches for the different situations in which you find yourself reflecting, and for the differing purposes for reflecting in the first place. It is important for you to build up a 'kit-bag' of reflective strategies, some formal, others less so, as ways of learning from your practice and experiences throughout your course. One strategy is not necessarily appropriate for all situations. As a result, this chapter and the next explore the very practical aspects of reflecting, enabling you to select from different approaches depending on the context in which you are reflecting and what you want to achieve from it.

Most reflection will be done on your own. Reflection is a solitary learning activity and, while other people can help you to do it, the insights and learning that are achieved will be just yours. The ways in which you achieve these, however, can be many and varied. It is worth remembering that, just as there are many routes and means of transport to get yourself from A to B, there are also many strategies that you can use for reflection. The purpose of building a reflective practice skill set is that the techniques, strategies and approaches become part of the way you are as a practitioner – reflection becomes automatic, so much so that unless you stop to think about it, it is embedded in your professional persona.

WORKING WITH YOUR LEARNING STYLE

In Chapter 2 you worked through the activity of identifying your learning style. We ended that section by presenting a table of the learning activities that suit each particular style (Table 2.4, p. 53). We want to return to this briefly, so that you can begin to think about the types of reflective strategy that will most suit your style, and actively work to develop this. A word of caution, though – as with all diagnostic and labelling tools, this one is only meant to give you an insight, and some ideas about how you can use the tendencies identified. Just because you appear to 'fit' mostly into one preferred learning style or another does not mean that you need to try to alter who and what you are. Nor does it mean that you necessarily operate from that basis at all times, as everyone is a mixture of all the features. Your preferred learning style, therefore, is where most of your tendencies lie, based on the answers you gave on the day that you completed the questions. This does not mean that you are fixed in this, nor that you cannot work to move consciously from one style to another.

Reflective activity

You've now had some time between identifying your learning style in Chapter 2 and working with it through Chapters 3 and 4. So perhaps it's a good time to reflect back on your reactions to doing that activity and what you might have discovered about yourself.

Firstly, did the preferred learning style category that you fell into provide any shocks? Did you have a mental picture of the category that you would have liked to have been in? Were these the same? If not, has falling into a different category made you think at all about:

● your perception of yourself

● the ways in which you go about your learning?

Secondly, look back at Table 2.4 on p. 53 and consider the types of activity suggested for your learning style. How many of these would you consciously say were 'you'? How many did you read and think 'No, I wouldn't want to do that'?

Now scan the activities suggested for the other learning styles. How many of these appeal to you as well?

You should now have a list of the types of activity you can plan to use that will suit your learning style, and therefore engage your interest and motivation. All of these can be used actively within reflective practice, so keep this list at hand and plan to incorporate some of these activities when you reflect by yourself.

KEY POINTS

● Being aware of your learning style enables you to select the methods for learning through reflection that will suit you most

● Planning your reflective learning through different kinds of activity will maintain your interest and maximize your learning from your experiences

---

THINKING THINGS OVER

Much of the reflection that you do will be inside your head. It is here that the distinction between reflection-in-action and reflection-on-action will become most apparent.

Reflection-in-action

We cannot be aware of our thought and decision-making processes every time we do something – at the very least we wouldn't get anything done! But, there are times when we are aware of consciously thinking about alternatives to action and actively selecting from them while we are doing it. For instance, you may be having a conversation with a patient but at the same time thinking 'What's going on here?', 'What might be the reason for this?' or 'What is the best way of dealing with this?'

When you start in your practice placements, you will probably be more aware of reflecting-in-action because the situations will be unfamiliar. As a result you will have to work hard at understanding what is going on and have to think through many of your actions before you do them. Take, for instance, what Kim says in the following case study.

Case study

Kim's experience

Kim is a 25-year-old second year midwifery student working a placement with the community midwife. This incident happened during an antenatal clinic at the GP surgery, where wall mounted sphygmomanometers were used routinely. Kim was used to using electronic ones in the obstetric unit, but was aware that she needed to be proficient at taking blood pressure readings with traditional equipment although it was much harder.

"I was going to take Mrs Goode's blood pressure. She is a large lady in her fifth pregnancy and had previously suffered from high blood pressure while pregnant. I knew it was important to get an accurate reading, but also that the only equipment available was a wall mounted sphyg. While placing the cuff around her upper arm I noticed that it wasn't big enough to fit around her arm. I didn't know whether a larger was available at the surgery so I made the decision to continue with the one I had. When I inflated the cuff the Velcro fastening began to rip and eventually the cuff came flying off. Mrs Goode looked at me and made a comment about having 'fat arms'. I made light of the situation, apologized and went to find a larger cuff."

This is a simple example of reflecting-in-action. Unfortunately, Kim made an inappropriate decision, even though she had thought things through in the first place. Her decision-making was flawed as she was not thinking in the best interests of the patient or in clinical terms about obtaining the most accurate reading, but in terms of inconvenience.

You will often find yourself reflecting-in-action, and it is worth making a mental note of those occasions so that you are aware that you are practising reflectively. What is harder is recognizing when you are practising in a routine way, or do things because you are told to do them without thinking. It is very easy, especially as a beginning practitioner, to allow feelings of insecurity and wanting to fit in to influence the actions you take, rather than actually stopping to think about whether these are the best courses of action to take. A cue for you to stop and think is when you feel uncomfortable about doing what others have asked you to do, or when you are aware that things are being done in a way that is incorrect.

Reflecting-in-action in this way contributes to 'thoughtful' practice, or the ways that responsible practitioners think in action. It is what, to some extent, identifies professional practitioners from unqualified staff, as they are constantly sifting through alternatives in their head to determine the best and most appropriate care. Most reflecting-in-action is done unconsciously, or without us being aware of it. It becomes the way that practitioners practise automatically (Rolfe *et al.*, 2011). But initially, by being aware of doing this, you will not only be taking steps to becoming a professional practitioner but you are more likely to make the most appropriate decisions for your patients.

Over to you

Next time you are in practice, talk to your supervisor, or any other person you are working with, about the way that they use reflection-in-action. You may find that you need to explain what you are talking about first, as many practitioners may not be aware of the theoretical concept of reflection-in-action. However, once you explain, it is more than likely that they will know exactly what you are talking about and can give you plenty of examples of the ways in which they use reflection-in-action throughout their working day.

Reflecting-in-action helps to safeguard against practice that has become routine and leads us towards conscious awareness of our actions and decisions. It is the way in which we can deliver individualized, rather than generalized, care that is tailored to the unique needs of each patient. What it can also do is provide us with the material for reflecting-on-action.

Reflection-on-action

Reflection-on-action is the process we are more likely to be aware of when we are reflecting. It occurs after the event, rather than as it is happening (see Chapter 1 for a definition). Reflection-on-action is the main way you will be using reflective practice overtly throughout your course, as you reflect by yourself, with and for others.

Reflecting-on-action as a thoughtful activity may happen quite spontaneously, or be something that you take time to do deliberately. Either way, there is a difference between using the reflective cycle to explore experiences and simply thinking them over in your head.

When we use reflective practice, we are reflecting for two main purposes:

● To learn from the experience
● To frame action that we will take.

These two features differentiate active reflection-on-action from the mulling over that goes on in our heads most of the time, which is mistakenly considered by many practitioners to be reflective practice. You may hear other people say that they 'do' reflective practice all the time, but what they really mean is that they think about what they are doing. Reflective practice as a conscious activity is a great deal more than that, as you will have already come to realize.

Deliberate reflection-on-action helps us to develop our understanding of situations so we can learn from them and change our future practice. When we create time to do this we are choosing to use our time to make sense of our experiences.

There's more to reflective practice
than you may think.

Time is a valuable resource for most of us, and therefore deserves to be put to good use. So, when you do set aside time to reflect, it is worth ensuring that you plan to use it effectively and for some purpose.

Most of the activities you have met so far in this book have asked you to engage in some sort of reflection by using cue questions. The purpose of this was to start you reflecting without the mystique and aura of it being 'reflective practice'. Hopefully, by now you will have realized that there are many different ways of reflecting, and not all of them are confined to structures and strategies. You can learn just as much from purposefully thinking issues through, provided you identify the learning and take some action as a result. However, you can also learn by working through a framework for reflection, and when you start out in reflective practice this might be a way of organizing both the reflective processes and your thoughts. Once you understand what it is you are trying to achieve, and plan to use the reflective mechanisms to do this, it will become second nature.

So, how do we do it? This is more difficult to help you with, for the simple reason that, if we provide you with examples, it becomes written reflection, which is dealt with in the next section! What we can do, though, is to show you how others use contemplative reflection-on-action to make sense of their experiences, and hope that this will provide you with clues as to how you can use it yourself. The other way is to go back to your preferred learning style and ask yourself how you can incorporate reflection-on-action within that.

Case study

Kim's experience (continued)

Do you remember Kim's experience when taking Mrs Goode's blood pressure? As well as reflecting-in-action, she made a point of thinking things through more deeply later on. The reasons she did this were that:

- She was embarrassed that she had caused Mrs Goode distress

- She realized that the procedure had not been effective

- She realized that she had made the wrong decision in choosing to carry on using the standard cuff.

- As she said:

"At the time I was thinking that the procedure would not be successful and I should stop using the cuff, but then part of me argued that there was maybe a chance that it would work and to wait for the outcome. I also knew we were under pressure to finish the clinic as we had a couple of home visits to do after clinic."

Kim used Johns' structured model of reflection to think her way through the incident and rationalize what she had done. She came to further understandings about it, and managed to see clearly where her priorities had been at that time. She was very concerned about the distress and embarrassment that she had caused Mrs Goode. She realized that it was this concern that prompted her to think about the way she delivered care, and that perhaps she had fallen into the trap of practising routinely rather than really thinking about what she was doing with each patient.

Her learning: Kim realized that the delivery of individualized care has to be a deliberate and considered activity, otherwise care is routine. She learned that sometimes she does not put the patient at the front of her care decisions and delivery.

Her action: She resolved to never make decisions based on time and inconvenience again. She vowed that she would try to look at patients' individual needs when delivering care.

This process took Kim about five minutes, as she was able to sit quietly during her coffee break after the incident and reflect on what had happened. Despite the fact that it took so little time, the understanding that Kim developed, and her resolve to change her actions, will have long-lasting consequences for her future practice.

Reflective activity of this sort need not take a lot of time, and a lack of time is no excuse for not thinking incidents and experiences over reflectively after they have occurred. It is not as though you will need to reflect in this way on everything that happens to you. But making reflection-on-action a habitual part of your practice will help you in developing your own knowledge and understanding for your practice. At the end of the day, it will probably actually save you time, because the learning achieved and the changes you make to your practice are immediate.

Over to you

Reflection-on-action in this way has to be a deliberate activity. You have to take the decision to do it – no-one can force you. So, it really is over to you this time! Will you rise to the challenge of trying to reflect on at least one incident or experience every day you are in practice?

KEY POINTS

- Reflection-in-action occurs as we are working, and is often unconscious
- By deliberately taking notice of when we are using reflection-in-action we will be aware of and maximize our learning
- Reflection-in-action can be seen as 'thoughtful practice'
- Reflection-on-action is a deliberate activity that occurs after the event
- We need to make time to use reflection-on-action by ourselves as thinking things over
- Getting into the habit of mentally reviewing and reflecting on experiences every day will begin the process of developing reflective practice
- Reflection-on-action is more than simply thinking about our practice
- Reflective practice is about identifying our learning and taking action as a result of using the ERA cycle

REFLECTIVE WRITING

The other way we can use the reflective processes within our learning is through writing reflectively. This has a different character and process from thinking things through reflectively and, although it is probably less prevalent in professional practice on a day-to-day basis, it is an extremely valuable way of learning from practice and becoming a consciously reflective practitioner. It is also a way that you will create evidence to convince others of your development.

Writing reflectively

As a student, you will be required to record much of your reflective activity. This may take various forms and formats, and these will often be provided for you, such as in reflective reviews, portfolio entries or essay formats exploring a particular incident or element of practice. So far you have met many different strategies and approaches to reflection in this book, from structured reflection through various different models to less formal, but just as valuable ways of reflective learning and uncovering knowledge. In this section we explore the value of written reflection, or deliberately using strategies of writing as a way of reflecting and learning from experience. This is, of course, used with any of the frameworks identified in Chapter 3, which will provide you with structures for ordering your thoughts and writing. Writing can be used to 'add value' to the reflective work you may do in your head, or with others.

What is reflective writing?

Reflective writing involves engaging in, and completing, the reflective cycle using writing processes to help you learn. **Reflective writing** differs from other forms of writing only in that it has one primary purpose – that of learning – to enable you to come to a different, or deeper, understanding of whatever you are reflecting on. The other results of writing, such as having a record of what you have done, or completing an assignment, are supplementary to this, and it is worth bearing this in mind when creating strategies for reflective writing for yourself – or, indeed, doing the actual writing.

Reflective writing
Writing for the purpose of learning from experience

Reflective activity

The last time you wrote

Think back to the last time you wrote a piece of academic work. Draw a line down the middle of your page. On the left hand side try to answer the following questions about what you wrote.

1 What did you write?

2 What was the purpose (why did you write it)?

3 How did you decide what, and what not, to write?

4 How did you decide on the order of what you wrote?

5 How did you organize or structure what you wrote?

On the right hand side of the page try to think about the 'why' questions – why were you writing, why did you include some things and leave others out? Why did you order it in this way? Why did you organize what you were writing in this way?

Now, try to think more deeply about the process of writing itself and what was going on while you were writing. Did the act of writing as a mental activity enable other things to happen? For instance, if you were writing an essay, did you find that you were drawing conclusions that you didn't realize you had reached? If you were writing a reflective review, did you remember things in the descriptive stage that you had previously forgotten? If you were writing a report on a client, did you start to make connections between things that you hadn't seen before?

Finally, what, for you, makes the process of writing different from the processes used in thinking things over in your head?

We asked you to think about what happened as a result of the process of your writing – whether you added something to your work that wasn't previously there, or whether you began to see something in a different light as a result of writing. This provides an illustration of the transformative nature of writing when viewed from the *writing-to-learn* perspective (Allen *et al.*, 1989) – the act of writing in itself adds to the way in which we view our experiences. We can actively plan to use this feature of writing when we choose to write reflectively.

Transformative
Changing or developing the ways in which we see things

Features of reflective writing

Reflective writing can be seen as building on and developing the skills that we already have in other forms of writing. When using reflective writing, we might think about the following features.

The reason we are writing

We always write for some purpose, even if it is simply a note reminding someone to get the washing in if it rains. Not only is writing purposeful, it is also deliberate – we have to decide to write, and give all of our attention to it at the time, as few thoughts, other than very simple things such as 'Do I need another cup of coffee?' can be going on in our heads at the same time. This combination of thinking, and translating those thoughts into writing, involves complex mental and physical processes that force us to focus completely on what we are doing. When we decide to write reflectively, we need to create the time and space to do so, as with any other type of writing; in other words, we make a commitment of our time and energy to the writing. Writing reflectively is a deliberate strategy to commit ourselves to identifying our learning, and framing action as a result. The consequences of this are that when we write we make a commitment to both the content and process of what we are writing. When writing reflectively this commitment becomes all important, in that we need a stimulus or a purpose for doing it and very often this arises from within ourselves and our practice.

How we can use writing to help order our thoughts

Secondly, writing forces us to impose some sort of order on the content of what we are writing. The order for some reflective writing will be given to you by the lecturers you are writing for as part of your course, by a reflective model or perhaps by a portfolio structure. For less formal writing, however, you have the freedom to write in whatever way you want, because the writing only needs to make sense to yourself.

The process of writing helps us to find both a structure for its content and an order for the points we want to make. Therefore, it also helps us to prioritize and identify what is important and what is not within the writing. How does this work? One reason is that our writing speed is limited by our typing speed or how fast we can physically write. This is slower than the speed at which we think, therefore we are slowed down in our thinking as we mentally sift and segregate the most important things to write. We cannot write at the speed we think, or even at the speed we talk; thus writing reflectively will be very different in content and structure from the way we reflect when talking to others or by ourselves contemplatively. It has three distinct features that can be seen as an advantage:

- We are forced to acknowledge issues that may be ignored if we are carrying on a conversation or reflecting inside our heads
- We can put a hierarchical order to issues that are significant to us
- This enables us to work through these issues as we have identified them, rather than being side-tracked into other things.

These make reflective writing an extremely personal process, and one that helps us work systematically through a process of reflection.

This differs from simply thinking things through, where we may get stuck going round and round in circles in our head.

The purpose of creating a permanent record

Although this point may seem obvious, writing creates a permanent record that can be returned to and reconsidered. It is important because:

- **It helps to provide a fuller picture of what has gone on.** The act of writing helps us to remember not only things we think we have forgotten but also things that may be hidden or overlaid by others that take priority. In trying to recall things that have happened to us and recount them verbally, we are selective in what we remember – the problem of hindsight bias. Very often we are convinced that we have remembered every detail, yet others who were also there at the time might say 'Yes, but do you remember this too...' Thus writing will jog our memory and fill in another piece of the jigsaw puzzle.

- **In writing things down we record what our memory allows us to remember at the time.** This might be close to the event, or at some time distant. This creates at least one account of the event, which can be used in the future for reflective activity. This original description can act as a memory jogger the next time you read it when more, or different, details and explanations of what has happened occur to us.

- **The written record allows us to put the event away and return to it at a later date.** As a result of the time and space created we may take a different perspective on the event and see it in a different way, by filling in more information or considering it in the light of new or alternative experiences and knowledge.

● **In writing things down we cannot ignore or forget them.** Rolfe *et al.* provide the anecdote of one student who said that:

> *An advantage in writing things down was that it made you deal with them, unlike being able to ignore them if they are in your head. He said that once they had appeared on paper there was a constant reminder and this acted as a prompt to sort them out, and that to some extent this was a hidden effect of writing – that it acted as a conscience so that you couldn't conveniently forget things – that they may turn out to be the key to a problem that you haven't yet found.*

Rolfe et al., 2011, p. 66

How we can be creative through writing

Writing in itself can be creative. How often have you sat down with the intention of writing one thing and ended up with something completely different? This is why many academic tutors suggest that the introduction to a piece of written work is the last part to be written – so that you can ensure you introduce the work you are presenting, and not the work you intended to write! Our mind takes us down paths as a result of considering the material in front of us at that particular time – it helps us create an alternative, and sometimes unexpected, sense of what we are seeing. Thus we may make connections between pieces of information that in the past we had not contemplated. The writing process helps us to *integrate* disparate information sets into new combinations, enabling us to take a different perspective on an issue. Writing may lead to creative thinking, where not only can you justify and defend your actions, but develop new understandings and perspectives on a situation, or come to understand a past event in a different light.

Using writing to develop our analytical skills

One of the effects of increasing the amount of writing we do is that we get more used to being analytical in how we do it. It really is one of those things that gets easier the more you do! Initially, when you start writing reflectively you will probably find that you want the structure provided for you by some sort of a reflective framework. However, as you get used to ordering the different elements in your head, and reviewing your experiences through the reflective processes, you will find that you start to experiment with the frameworks or decide to omit some stages as you go along. You may find you adapt a framework to make it 'fit' more closely with the type of experience you are reflecting on, or the purpose you want to fulfil. You may even end up creating your own framework, especially if you move beyond the confines of using only critical incidents, into using reflective practice in a predictive way.

When we analyze, we break things down into their component parts. We learn to see those components as separate elements and consider their role in relation to the whole. Some parts will be more important, or significant, for what we are learning than others. The features of writing that we have already identified, for creating a permanent record and providing an order to our thoughts, also aid us in becoming more analytical. They do this by giving us the means to break things down through a framework or specific structure that the experience itself did not possess. We record the experience descriptively, as we perceived it. We then analyze our description by identifying and building on the separate features of it. The written record provides us with a way of slowing this process down, as our fingers try to keep up with our brain. This, in turn, makes us stop and think differently, or more deeply. This is in contrast to when we sit and think things through without writing, as there are no mental stops where we say 'What am I going to write next?' or 'What did that really mean?' or 'Did I really say that?'

Using writing to develop our critical thinking

Within the reflective cycle, being critical about our experiences follows on from the analytical stages. By this we do not mean finding fault or being negative, but taking an objective stance to exploring something in a balanced way. Many writers see the reflective process as key to developing critical thinking, and reflective writing as a crucial process of enabling it to happen. Critical thinking is also regarded as crucial to the ways in which practitioners make decisions about their practice.

critical thinking
The processes involved in exploring and weighing up possibilities for action and making a rational choice

The notion of critical thinking has been the subject of much debate, but one of the most recent definitions is that it is:

> The gathering, sifting, synthesizing and evaluating of information which enables the practitioner to act as a knowledgeable doer – someone who selects, combines, judges and uses information in order to proceed in a professional manner.
>
> *Price and Harrington, 2010, p. 8*

So, critical thinking is about weighing up all the possibilities for action and being able to make a reasoned and rational choice. Brookfield (1987) has identified the features of people who are critical thinkers as:

- engaging in productive and positive activity
- viewing their thinking as a process rather than an outcome
- varying in their manifestations of critical thinking according to context
- experiencing triggers to critical thinking as positive or negative
- feeling comfortable with the emotive as well as the rational elements of the critical thinking process.

So how can reflective writing help us to become critical thinkers? If we think back to the processes of the reflective cycle, we can see that in choosing to adopt these we will automatically be working in the ways that critical thinkers work. Brookfield (1987) defines the components of critical thinking as:

- **Identifying and challenging assumptions:** This means ensuring that you write down the assumptions you made in relation to an event you describe. These assumptions may be the knowledge or theory you used, or particular paradigm cases you remember, or experiential learning.

- **Recognizing the importance of context:** Our actions are never context-free – we all work within the confines of our experiences of the world, time and places we have lived. These ultimately interfere with and affect the way in which we see others. Exploring the context of events and acknowledging the limitations of our perceptions enables us to think more analytically, and therefore critically. Writing these down provides us with a way of objectifying our experiences; we are able to stand outside the experiences as personal and view them from a different perspective.

- **Exploring and imagining alternatives:** Critical thinking involves being able to compare and evaluate different solutions to problems, or consider events in order to uncover new and different ways of perceiving the world. Writing enables us to explore and imagine alternative viewpoints by providing us with structures and questions which challenge our previous way of looking at things.

- **Reflective scepticism:** Being sceptical protects us from accepting 'universal truths', 'common sense' or that there is only ever one explanation for an event or one way of looking at it. Developing scepticism leads us to question and seek alternative answers – it may lead ultimately to the development of new understandings by encouraging us to reject previously accepted explanations.

Each of these is incorporated within the reflective cycle; hence, in choosing to write reflectively, we will also be developing our powers of critical thinking.

Using writing to develop new understandings and knowledge

The processes of writing can help develop our understanding of what we are experiencing, and may lead us to create new knowledge for ourselves. This can happen at any stage of the reflective cycle because the very process of ordering the way we write things down may create a new way of seeing things or provide a new perspective.

Using writing to show that we understand something

We cannot write convincingly about things that we do not understand. By being able to write about them we show ourselves that we can explain it and understand it. How often have you tried to explain something to someone else, and at the end realized that you knew more than you thought you did?

Or conversely, how often have you found yourself rambling through an explanation for something and ending up confusing your listener even more because you hadn't really got the important points straight in your head? Writing also has this effect. If you can write a clear description and analysis of the experience you are reflecting on, it will provide you with more clarity about it. You will cut out all the extraneous information and focus, in the end, on the key elements for your learning and action for practice.

Writing in the first person

If we are writing about things that have happened to us personally, or in relation to ourselves, it is obvious that we need to write in the first person. This means writing using 'I'. This makes us take responsibility for our part in the experience, and acknowledge our role in what has happened. It also helps to avoid blaming other people for what happened, because their part will be located in the descriptive part of the account. The purpose of reflective writing is personal (usually); therefore, it is our own behaviour that needs to be the focus of the writing. It is clearly nonsense to try to write reflectively in the third person, or to take yourself out of your account. Equally, it is unreasonable to try to change the behaviour of others, so try to avoid saying 'They should have …' clearly, they didn't, and it isn't your concern, other than as a point of learning.

Reflective activity

Take some time to think about what you have just read about the nature of reflective writing and how it is different from thinking things through.

How does this, as a reflective strategy, interlink with your preferred learning style?

Can you identify an example from your practice that you could consider using written reflection rather than thoughtful reflection? What might be the advantages of one method of reflection over the other?

The features of writing are significant for how we learn. But writing reflectively involves more than simply 'writing things down': it often involves the analysis and identification of the roles we have played in events in our lives. But this depends on what we are reflecting on and the purpose we want the reflection to achieve. Just as reflective writing as a whole can be used in different ways by people with different learning styles, it is important to remember that no one strategy will suit everyone. Equally, there is no right and wrong about reflective writing and the adoption of a technique contrary to your own personality, learning style and inclination is likely to be doomed to failure from the start. In the next section we present a selection of ways that you can use to write reflectively.

KEY POINTS

● Reflective writing is writing that is done for the purpose of learning

● Reflective writing builds on the unique features of writing in creating artefacts that can be used

● Reflective writing can be used within any of the preferred learning styles

STYLES AND STRATEGIES FOR REFLECTIVE WRITING

Rolfe *et al.* (2011) suggest that strategies for writing can be divided into two main types – analytical and creative. This section uses and expands this classification to provide you with a range of examples and illustrations. Some of these you will have met already – either through the examples given in this book or because you are required to use them in your course. But others will not be so familiar to you, in fact, you may not even have considered them as useful strategies for reflective writing at all.

Analytical strategies

These are called analytical strategies because the processes of analysis and synthesis are incorporated within the process of writing. They are the ones that you will meet most commonly because they are amenable to use within the reflective frameworks that have come to dominate reflective practice. They are also likely to use most of the stages of the ERA reflective cycle, although at first the movement to the third stage, that of taking action, is likely to remain at the 'framing action' level. The purpose of these strategies is to incorporate 'stepping back' from an incident and taking an objective view of it. The end result is often a piece of writing that attempts to be balanced and evaluative of all features of the experience or event. It is these strategies that are most likely to be directed by others, required as coursework and seen by others. Hence the purpose is to demonstrate your learning in having achieved the required outcomes. This makes them amenable to assessment through objective marking criteria, and enables students' assignments to be compared with each other.

Learning journals

This is an umbrella term that incorporates diaries, learning logs, progress files and records of achievement. Learning journals may also be called 'portfolios', or be part of a portfolio. A learning journal's essential characteristics are:

● It is compiled on an incremental basis over a period of time.

● It is focused on identifying learning that has occurred.

● It provides a record of events and experiences.

● It contains reflective commentaries or accounts.

Journal writing is where many students start their journey of reflective writing, as it is often a required course component. For this reason, learning journals are often structured through a reflective framework, and students are required to build up a portfolio of these throughout their course or a particular module.

Other models for learning journals can be found when they are used to create a written record of activity in practice, for instance, or in relation to reviewing specific learning achievements. An example of this is presented in the extract below. Tim was a student on a multidisciplinary module on critical reflection.

Case study

Tim's learning journal

Tim is a mature student embarking on a career change from being a local government officer in the special educational needs section. He has started the osteopathy programme, which will last four years, and will result in registration with the British Osteo-pathic Council as an independent practitioner.

"Today's session was exploring reflective writing. I must admit that I was a bit sceptical about this because I had not really thought about writing reflec-tively at all. My starting point was that I considered 'writing' to be something that I had to do for other people – reports at work, case notes, academic work – and didn't see writing as something for myself at all. I also saw it as beyond my control: we have to write for other people most of the time. Also, I tend to be a bit phased by all the rules about writing. As a result of all of this lot I suppose I have not thought about writing as a way that I can learn for myself.

The session led us through a series of what I can only call 'eye-opening' exercises. We looked, in pairs and in groups, at our experiences and attitudes towards writing, and why we thought about it the way we did. We were also challenged by the facilitator to try to think differently about writing. Several people presented examples of how they had used writing in ways that I had never thought about, such as decision-making and poetry writing. Another novel idea was the idea of two people writing a dialogue, or using a running journal to keep notes on the development of a case.

I learned a great deal, although I didn't expect to. The main learning for me was that I am in a rut in the way I think. I can see the opportunities that reflective writing can present, and will definitely start to keep a learning journal from now on. Even if it is only as simple as this entry, it will provide a record of my progress on the course, and document my achieve-ments for me. So, three things that I have learned today are:

- I can use writing as a way of learning.

- Writing can be under my control.

- Reflective writing does not have to be restricted to a particular format – I can create my own to suit my purposes."

If you are required to keep a learning journal as part of your course, the structure and components for it have probably been supplied for you. If you do not have to do this, it is worth thinking about keeping a journal anyway, as a record of your progress during the course.

The types of thing that you could put into it are:

- a reflective write-up of each day
- an evaluation of your educational experiences
- a reflective review of your learning from practice encounters
- specific critical incident analyses of events that have happened
- your planning for the future as a result of your reflections
- any of the work that you have done in response to the reflective activities in this book.

It is useful to incorporate some physical structure in your journal that allows you to return to the entry, re-read and annotate it with further thoughts. One way of doing this is to start a new page for each entry and write the description of the incident on the left-hand page, the right-hand page being dated for the reflective analysis and writing. This enables you to return to the entry on future occasions and add further reflections to it. This will also document your changing perspective on the event, as you learn to see it in different ways with the passing of time and more experiences.

Another useful tip is, as Tim has done, to try to identify three things that you have learned from each day, experience or journal entry.

In this way the journal becomes a dynamic organism, and many people come to regard them as essential to the ways in which they make sense of the world. In fact, one student's learning journal seemed to acquire a personality all of its own and she began to refer to it as 'her'! Just creating the physical space and time to review and record what has happened during a day provides a means of tying up loose ends and creating closure for things that have happened. Learning journals also provide us with a mechanism for acknowledging our learning and progress, and help us to put events into a wider perspective.

Over to you

What are your thoughts about the idea of keeping a learning journal?

Are you open to the challenge of trying it for a week and evaluating its use at the end of that time?

Even if you do decide that journal keeping is not for you, complete the reflective cycle by writing up the experience and file it in your portfolio as a learning experience.

Critical incident analyses

In this book we have used this term to refer to any specific occurrence that happens to us that we can use as a focus for reflective activity. Utilizing these for analysis using a structured framework enables us to build up a collection of evidence of our learning and development. Many of the case studies throughout this book are critical incident analyses written by students for particular reasons. Few have been presented in their entirety, because of their length and because they have been used to illustrate specific aspects of reflective practice. The following account, however, is a complete critical incident analysis.

Case study

Solomon

Solomon is a 30-year-old phlebotomist working in elderly-care in a large district general hospital

Critical incident analysis "I was working as a phlebotomist in a busy acute and elderly care directorate, which consisted of six wards (approximately 150 patients). It was my job to take all the routine blood samples from the patients using venepuncture. I was already halfway through my designated patients and was well ahead of time. If I completed all my work I was permitted to go home early. This was on my mind as I entered the room of a lady in her early 70s who had been admitted with dehydration. At the time, it was this particular directorate's policy that phlebotomists were required to wear gloves at all times when taking blood. However, there was a shortage of high-sensitivity gloves, so often we were forced to use standard gloves. This made palpating a vein and feeling for a pulse more difficult.

I spoke to the patient, telling her what I was about to do, and she reassured me that this was quite routine for her. After applying the tourniquet and palpating what I believed to be one of the digital cephalic veins in the back of the patient's hand, I proceeded to cleanse the area and entered the vein using a butterfly needle. Almost immediately I noticed an unusual amount of swelling around the puncture site, and so I removed the tourniquet, applied direct pressure to the site and removed the needle. The swelling had increased to about the size of half a table tennis ball in the matter of a few seconds. At this point I decided that the needle had penetrated both sides of the vein and had nicked one of the underlying arteries. After about five minutes, the swelling began to disperse, and so I removed the pressure and observed the wound for another few minutes to ensure that the bleeding had stopped. I then applied a dressing and checked her condition. The patient assured me that she felt fine and was in no pain. I then approached the nurse in charge of the bay and informed her that I might have nicked an artery in the lady's hand but that the swelling had stopped and that she was not otherwise affected. I re-checked the patient's condition before leaving the ward and she seemed to be in good spirits."

Reflection "In this instance, my main objective was to take blood from this patient as quickly as possible. I wanted to complete my round swiftly to enable me to finish work early. However, once the incident had occurred my priorities changed so that my aim was to stop this woman's arterial bleeding. I then wanted to ensure that the relevant people knew about what had happened to enable them to take appropriate action.

The reason that I intervened in the way that I did was to prevent any more haemorrhaging. The application of direct pressure was the method I was taught to slow down or to stop bleeding. Informing the staff nurse enabled her to inform the doctor that the blood had not been taken. It also allowed them to observe the area in case of any complications.

As far as complications for the patient were concerned, there were very few to note. There was a slight bruising of the area, combined with some minor swelling. The wound healed satisfactorily within a few days. The family was informed of the incident by the nursing staff after one of them noticed the bruise on the lady's hand, but they were satisfied with the explanation given, so they did not complain. They stated that they were pleased that the patient was making a recovery and that there was no harm done to the patient herself. Professionally speaking, the only consequence suffered by myself was a verbal reprimand from my superior for damaging the lady's artery. However, I informed her that the main reason for this happening in the first place was the lack of proper equipment, i.e. high sensitivity gloves. This was not the first time that this complaint had been aired, and it was again brought to the attention of the senior nurse manager of the directorate. Because there had actually been an incident involving a patient this time, the guidelines for venepuncture were changed. My feelings at the time of the occurrence were varied. The main emotion was one of fear: fear for the patient's well-being as well as fear for the consequences that I might suffer, for example, an official reprimand or other disciplinary action. Before I entered the room, I had been confident of my skills and abilities within that environment. I had carried out this procedure hundreds of times before without any significant difficulties. Once this happened, I felt exactly the opposite of this. There was almost a surge of panic flowing through me – while this may have been an overreaction, it is what I felt, possibly because I had been so confident beforehand.

The patient's reaction to the incident was very good. Indeed, she dealt with it better than I did. I had been speaking with her while the swelling was going down in her hand, and she seemed quite calm. After I had completed my round, I returned to check on her condition, and she seemed to be quite happy. She was sitting with her visitors, laughing and joking. I saw her the next day and asked her how her hand was and she informed me that she had forgotten about the whole episode. This reassured me that her hand was fine and that she suffered no emotional trauma due to this situation."

Influencing factors "The main internal factor that influenced my actions at the beginning of the incident was my impatience. My biggest concern was that I was held up with the patient and so would not finish my workload early. As it was the weekend and the weather was pleasant, I did not want to spend any more time than was necessary at work. After I had scratched the woman's artery, the factor that influenced my actions was the training I had received beforehand, combined with a newfound sense of urgency arising from the panic that I was experiencing. I also believe that overconfidence was a major contributing factor in my initial actions. I had a fair degree of previous experience and had never had a problem like this one before.

The external factors that were affecting me included the patient and the equipment that I was using to take the blood. The patient had informed me that the back of her hand was the place where other phlebotomists were usually successful at drawing blood. As the woman had been admitted with dehydration, I was inclined to believe her. From past experience, I found that the hand was usually easier to palpate than the crook of the elbow, although research tends to suggest the opposite. The equipment influenced my actions, because the gloves that I was wearing were not suited to the type of work being performed, and so were, in themselves, a contributing factor.

The knowledge base for my actions was the training that I had received during purpose-designed study days, including a practical course in venepuncture. Another source of knowledge for reacting in the way that I did was some basic first-aid knowledge from other courses that I had attended. These courses taught me how to deal with a patient with arterial bleeding. The last source of knowledge was the practical experience that I had in taking venous blood samples. I had been taking blood from patients for over a year with no major difficulties, and had become quite proficient."

Alternative actions "I believe that I could have dealt with the initial situation better. My actions after the situation had occurred, however, were directly in accordance with the guidelines laid out by that Trust.

My other choices could have included making an attempt to take blood from a different part of the woman's hand or arm. I could also have attempted to palpate the area without gloves on and marked the best area to make an attempt. I do not think that this would have made a significant difference, though. As the lady was dehydrated, it is reasonable to assume that her blood pressure would have been lower than normal. This would suggest that it would have been difficult to feel a pulse in her hand, particularly as this artery was situated below another blood vessel."

Learning "The only reasonable explanation as to my actions was my over-confidence in my abilities combined with my impatience in wanting to finish my shift early. This led to me not giving my full attention to the task at hand. This has led me to develop more patience in my work, and has also developed my attention span by making me think more about what I am doing when performing any procedure.

My feelings about the experience are varied. There is shocked realization that I was capable of making such a mistake in the first place, as well as the knowledge now that emergencies can happen at any time. I have also experienced a feeling of relief that it has happened, because it has led me to be more careful and pay attention in even the most routine of procedures.

The fact that the only consequence that I suffered was a verbal reprimand confirms to me that I followed the correct course of action. I followed the correct procedures as laid down by the Trust and was therefore covered legally. This shows that the procedures are in place for a reason, and that they should be followed at all times."

Use of a reflective framework "My overall conclusion is that the use of reflective practice is essential to the delivery of quality care. The above example shows how a formal layout of reflection allows us to look back on what we have done and learn from any outcomes. The main lessons included the correct use of time management and the importance of patience when carrying out all duties in a clinical environment. It has also demonstrated that it is through reflection that procedures change and are improved upon, in this instance the use of gloves in this particular directorate."

NB. References to published sources have been deleted from the original account to make it easier to read.

In this account the student clearly identifies how he has arrived at his conclusions in using critical incident analysis through a structured framework. He also acknowledges his learning from the incident and has framed action as a result of this experience. He chose to use a framework, in this case Johns' model of structured reflection, to guide his reflection, and clearly found this useful in helping him to identify his learning and future action.

Dialogical writing

In **dialogical** writing, the writer constructs a **hypothetical** conversation between themselves and another person. This could take the form of a question and answer session, or a developmental dialogue.

It is particularly useful where an experience has caused a negative emotional response and the writer needs to be able to stand back from the event and adopt a more analytical and cognitive understanding of the situation. Borton's extended framework is appropriate as a guide for dialogical writing,

Dialogical
Like a conversation/ dialogue

Hypothetical
Imaginary/possible

as it enables the account to be structured through a series of questions. Alternatively, it is useful to create a purpose-made structure for each event, dependent on the learning to be achieved, as in the following account.

Case study

Dialogical writing

Carl is a 35-year-old adult field nursing student

What is my previous experience? "I have worked for the last 16 years as a Royal Navy Medical Assistant and after my initial training period I further specialized as a Commando trained medic. This then led me to work almost exclusively with the Royal Marines, providing medical support for them on operations and exercises worldwide. Very often I would be the only medically trained person available for these men and further support from the Medical Officer and other medical staff would be a considerable distance away (if, indeed, they were even in the same country). I would provide this medical cover for up to 150 men in very isolated environments and as such I have had to become a medic competent in being able to work alone, not only in dealing with day to day coughs and colds but also in life-threatening immediate/emergency care such as trauma. I have had to work alone and in isolation from other medical staff, making decisions that have made the difference between life and death."

Why is this relevant to this incident? "This will hopefully explain why as a first-year student nurse I would be deemed competent enough by my mentor to be entrusted with immediate postoperative nursing care (although I should state that during this period my mentor was within the same nursing bay and was immediately available to me if I encountered any problems)."

What happened? "The patient at the centre of this incident was a 23-year-old lady who was admitted to the ward for a planned surgical incision and drainage of a pilonidal sinus. On admission this lady was in good health and was not suffering any other ailments of any description and her blood pressure was recorded at 118/72 millimetres of mercury (mmHg)."

What does this mean? Tortora and Grabowski (2003) describe blood pressure as the hydrostatic pressure exerted by blood on the artery walls as it flows through them and break the definition of blood pressure further into systolic blood pressure and diastolic blood pressure. Systolic pressure is the pressure exerted on the artery walls during systole (ventricular contraction), and in a young adult at rest this will rise to roughly 120mmHg. The diastolic pressure is the pressure on the artery walls during diastole (ventricular relaxation), which would be expected to be around 80 mmHg. This gives a normal value of approximately 120/80 mmHg for a young adult.

Go on "With these figures in mind I knew that on admission this patient had a relatively normal blood pressure. However on carrying out an initial check of this lady's baseline observations I was surprised to find that her blood pressure (which I checked manually with a sphygmomanometer and stethoscope) had dropped to 96/62 mmHg. Knowing this patient had just returned to the ward post-operation, from my previous experience I knew that a decreased systolic blood pressure was one of the signs of hypovolaemic shock."

So what did I do? "I wanted to check my patient's blood pressure again to make sure I had not misinterpreted my reading as the ward was busy and very noisy at this time; however, the reading I obtained was the same, so I informed the staff nurse, who immediately checked the patient's blood pressure for herself. The reading she obtained was similar to mine at 98/60 mmHg and was recorded as an early warning score which would trigger a managerial response. Before contacting the junior doctor we raised the foot of the bed to help the patient regain a normal blood pressure. On reporting these facts to the doctor (by phone as he was off the ward at the time) he agreed that the patient's blood pressure was lower than normal and he instructed the staff nurse to increase the drip rate of the intravenous infusion, which was still running through postoperatively. He also gave instructions for the staff nurse to inform him immediately if the patient's systolic blood pressure fell below 90mmHg and to check it every five minutes for the next 30 minutes and to continue with normal protocols if it began to rise. Thankfully our patient's blood pressure did start to rise and by two hours post-operation had returned to almost normal values."

So what was the problem? "I was very surprised that the staff nurse felt the need to request further advice from a doctor initially when simple nursing interventions could have improved our patient's blood pressure to the point where normal values might well have been achieved. What did surprise me was that the staff nurse did not act more positively on her own intuition although this could have been due to her own knowledge or experiences."

Now what sense can I make of this? "Internally my previous experience had a big effect on my actions, in that as an experienced Royal Navy medic I feel that I am quite competent to check a patient's blood pressure postoperatively. Externally I would have to seriously question my abilities/knowledge if I was unsure as to what action to take on finding a low blood pressure reading postoperatively given my previous employment. I realize, however, that the staff nurse has not had my experience and has been trained to work in different situations. I realize that I was judging her actions from my own knowledge base, and that this might not have been appropriate. She was responsible for the patient and followed her own reasoning in calling the doctor. Ultimately, it was up to the doctor to prescribe treatment. This was my problem, not hers."

Now what have I learned from this? "My main area of learning in light of my previous experience is that I would like to think that as a health care professional post-registration I will be able to carry out simple but effective and immediate nursing procedures to help improve a patient's outcome. However, seeing the staff nurse in this incident request further advice from a doctor before carrying out relatively simple nursing procedures has left me feeling that there are perhaps gaps within pre-registration nurse training. This whole incident has helped me to further my learning by showing me the relevance of checking blood pressure postoperatively, and by using the nursing process nurses can influence patient outcomes for the better. I have also realized that I am perhaps too quick to judge other people, especially as I have a different background from them. In a controlled ward situation I do not have the responsibility that I had in the field and maybe I need to learn to work in a team with the other health care professionals involved."

Reference

Tortora, G.J. and Grabowski, S.R. (2003) *Principles of Anatomy and Physiology,* 10th edn. John Wiley, New York.

This was an effective strategy for this reflective account because relatively few cue questions are used yet all stages of the ERA cycle are included. The use of the first person throughout enables the student to sort out his own feelings and responsibilities from those of the other person. It enabled him to let go of his judgement of the staff nurse and focus on the incident in terms of his own learning.

An advantage of this sort of writing is that the dialogue can be led by the writer themselves, in building up a logical sequence. In the account above the stages of the reflective process are all used, but in a way appropriate for the student. For instance, at the stage of exploring alternatives, the student thought about alternative explanations as opposed to alternative actions. His conclusions about the future relate to the way in which he views and assesses other people, and his awareness of making judgements in comparison with himself. His main learning outcome therefore arises not from anything to do with taking blood pressure (he had already recognized his competence in this), nor with the actions of the staff nurse, but from his own attitude to other people and his change of role now he is a student.

Making a case

Although similar to dialogical writing, the purpose of this strategy is to create an argument that will persuade another person of the value of the viewpoint presented. This is in many ways very close to an academic writing style, in that you need to present an analysis of a problem, its solutions and your proposals.

Creative strategies

These strategies are different from the analytical ones because they actively acknowledge the descriptive, personal and emotional components of experiences. In using these strategies, there is a recognition that, at times, we need to get beyond the immediate experience of the event, before we can free ourselves up to explore it analytically and reflectively. Rolfe *et al.* (2011, p. 88) call them creative because they involve 'using the imagination and transforming experience away from the rational ways of analysis which characterizes the above group and moves the writer into imagination and metaphor as a way of creating insight and facilitating learning'. The artefact produced may be deliberately one-sided or emphasize the emotionality of the writer's response as opposed to attempting to analyze within the narrative. This serves the purpose of helping the writer to overcome the initial responses to the situation by getting it down on paper in some way. The resulting piece can then be used as the focus for analysis and reflection, or discussion with another person.

It is unlikely that these types of reflective writing would be used in coursework for assessing students. However, they may be encouraged in testing out alternative ways of writing in exercises, or be included in students' private reflections on their learning. It would be extremely difficult to justify forcing a student to write in this way because of the vulnerability that can be exposed. It is worth remembering that anyone reading reflective writing will inevitably be making some sort of a judgement about what they are reading, and maybe about the person who has written it too. Indeed, as a student you should never be required to share writing of this kind with others. You are, of course, free to show it of your own volition, but you need to have thought carefully about the consequences of doing so.

Writing the unsent letter, memo or e-mail

The unsent letter, memo or e-mail all have the same effect – to clear the writer's head of the immediate emotions that accompany a distressing incident. This often occurs when we are angry with someone else or feel that a situation is out of our control, or that we are disempowered in some way.

The idea is that the writer writes exactly what they want to say to the other person involved in the event with no holds barred. Hence, the account may be very emotional, irrational and full of language that you wouldn't actually dream of using to the other person. The safety net is in the fact that the letter/memo/e-mail will not be sent – ever! This is a powerful way of bringing order to the chaos of a stressful situation, and serves the purpose of freeing up the brain to begin dealing with what has occurred. It provides distance from the event itself, yet enables the writer to stay in touch with what happened. Once the writer has got this all down on paper, the account is then used to deconstruct and reflect on what has happened. The result may well be a re-written letter or e-mail that is cleared of the emotionality of the original.

Many of the first accounts from new students resemble this type of work – although this is usually not intentional! For instance, the account below can be seen as an example of reflective writing that should never be made public.

Case study

The unsent letter

Felix is a 25-year-old first year nursing student on his first placement and is hoping to move into learning disabilities nursing at the end of this year. He writes:

Dear Sister

I was really angry at what I saw two trained nurses do today. Victor, an 86-year-old patient, had been vomiting faecal fluid for five days. Sarah, the staff nurse, was going to pass a nasogastric tube to relieve the pressure in his stomach. He had been left in a bed covered in vomit and appeared exhausted and upset. She left me with him while she went to get the equipment to pass the tube.

The tube was passed easily but I noticed that Victor was very anxious and put this down to the pain and discomfort he was feeling. Once in place the fluid was expected to drain from the tube, but this didn't happen, probably because the tube wasn't far enough into the stomach. Victor vomited, causing the tube to come out of his mouth. Sarah left the bay for another tube and to get more help. All the staff were busy, and as a result Victor was left lying in vomit for ten minutes waiting for the next shift to arrive. He looked completely exhausted and traumatized by the whole incident. Then it was decided that the nasogastric tube could wait until the following morning.

Due to the shift overlap handover, both nurses decided to change Victor's pyjamas swiftly. I was told to go off shift as I could be of no further use, but before doing so I noticed both nurses remove the pyjama top and replace it with a clean one without giving Victor a wash. No bathing, clean bed linen or mouth care was offered at all.

I felt absolutely dreadful at Victor's treatment, and pretty disgusted at the standards of care that I have witnessed on this ward. If these are the standards that you allow then I feel you should not be in charge. I certainly do not want to learn how to be a nurse from these qualified staff.

Yours sincerely

Felix

This was obviously a shocking incident as witnessed by a new student on his first placement. It clearly challenged Felix's beliefs and values about nursing, the care that patients can expect to receive and his faith in his mentor as a practitioner. Writing the incident down like this enabled Felix to pour out his feelings and emotions so he could then stand back from the incident. However, to make the incident public in this way would cause a great many more problems for Felix than it would solve. Hence he needed to reflect on what he had written and think about his own learning from the incident, and the implications for his future practice, rather than on the actions of the others involved. This is his reflective and analytical account.

Case study

Victor's treatment – a reflective and analytical account

"Reflecting back on the incident I feel annoyed and upset that I didn't do more at the time. This was my first ward and only my first week, which made me very unsure of my knowledge and expertise learned previously at the university. I lacked confidence, resulting in a breakdown of my communication skills. When Sarah, my mentor, left the bedside I am embarrassed to say I went numb, unable to speak. I just couldn't find any words appropriate to the situation and to comfort Victor.

When it came to the hygiene aspects of the incident I should have agreed to help but was unsure of how the nurses would react if I suggested a complete washdown and thorough changing of bedding and clothing. I was concerned with what and how they might feel towards me if I were to intervene."

Good points "It was very difficult at first to see any good points. I valued the educational input from Sarah. I have found the whole experience of reflecting on the incident an excellent learning tool and will use it in the future."

Bad points "Overall, there appears to be more negative points than positive ones. My communication skills appear lacking, which led to a breakdown in the nurse–patient relationship, resulting in an unprofessional standard of care. I feel that the patient was not central during the situation as his feelings were not considered throughout."

Analysis "Looking back over the incident I can now see why things turned out the way they did. Communication broke down between nurse and patient, and me and the nurse. Sarah and I were caught up in the teaching and learning aspect and were not concentrating on communicating with Victor. I later learned that Victor is hard of hearing. He must have been feeling very isolated, alone and confused as a result, which is why he got so distressed. Victor had also been given intramuscular metoclopramide to prevent nausea and vomiting. This can cause drowsiness, restlessness and depression – all shown by Victor at the time.

The problem with the insertion of the tube could have been avoided had Sarah measured the approximate distance from nose to stomach."

Victor's capacity to look after his own hygiene needs were severely restricted. He was unable to wash himself, change his clothes or his bedding. It was the nurses' responsibility to do this."

Conclusion

"Overall I feel that I should have been more assertive and got involved, despite my lack of experience. This does not excuse the overlooking of what should have been basic nursing care. If this situation happened again I would ensure that I communicated effectively with the patient and put his needs before my own. I would also ensure that I left the patient in a clean and comfortable condition, no matter whether that meant I was late going off shift."

The difference between these two accounts is clear. In the first Felix is incensed by the actions of others. In the reflective account he is able to focus on his own actions and identify his learning from the incident. Despite finding the whole event stressful, he has turned what was a negative event for all concerned into one that he has learned valuable lessons from for the future. He is also aware of his own values and standards regarding patient care, an uncomfortable awareness that his needs were given precedence over those of the patient, and that he needs to become more assertive.

The unsent memo and e-mail act in similar ways to this, they are simply another medium. However, there is just one word of caution with the unsent e-mail – it is far too easy to push the Send button!

Think twice before you hit the "send" button!

Writing to another person

Writing to another person is really a variation on the above strategy, but instead of imagining writing to the person involved in the event, the writer writes as if telling another person with whom they are familiar, be it a friend, a relative or even a respected teacher.

This technique enables the writer to put their own point of view, but this tends to be modified by the imagined effect on, or authority of, the recipient. It is more likely that this type of letter will include a description of what has happened, or it may include ideas and propositions from the writer that take a dialogue forward.

Writing as the other

With the technique of writing as the other, the writer attempts to put himself in the place of the other person in the event and tell the story from the other person's point of view. This can be useful in attempting to get someone to move beyond barriers that are preventing them from analyzing a situation, particularly if the writing is facilitated by using key questions. This can be supplemented by the writer writing of the event first from their own viewpoint and then from another's, or even from that of all the players in the interaction. While it is impossible to 'get inside someone else's head', the activity of attempting to see an event from a different point of view often enables insight to develop.

Writing as a journalist or outside observer

In the writing as a journalist or outside observer method the writer attempts to create a version of the incident as if they were merely observing, and not part of the action at all. It enables you to attempt to describe the incident from multiple viewpoints and has the effect of reducing the personal emotions involved.

Story telling

In story telling, the writer writes as if creating a story for an audience – either to be read aloud or to be read silently. In this way the unconscious thoughts that we were not aware of at the time of an experience can be brought to the fore and acknowledged. Metaphor can be used to recreate the experience, where the writer is able to impose his perspective on the account. Examples of this strategy may include giving the key players fictional names that reflect how the writer sees them, or imputing motives to players when they cannot have had access to this.

Poetry as reflective writing

Poetry can be seen in many ways as shorthand reflective writing, as each phrase or line is constructed to convey an image or concept. It is perhaps the archetypal style of creative writing, where the features of reflectively writing as having meaning for ourselves are most acutely obvious. Poetry is intensely personal, and is certainly not a strategy for everyone! However, many find it useful in helping them to work out their understandings of situations.

This intensely personal way of writing raises another issue that we need to consider when writing – that of how we establish safety for our writing.

Writing in safety

In order to feel comfortable with writing our reflections, we need to feel that we are in control of both the process and the outcomes of it. Here are a few issues to consider before you start writing.

Setting your own rules For reflective writing to serve the purpose of helping you to learn it is vital that you set the parameters or 'rules' for the writing, and that you are in control of the whole process.

Establishing the purpose of your reflection It is too easy to get into the habit of only reflecting on negative incidents, or using the reflective process simply for making sense of things in the past. Try instead to choose a selection of focuses for your reflective activity that involve thinking and planning for the future on the basis of what you need to learn and develop. You can use the learning opportunities identified in Chapter 4 as a checklist for this. Also, revisit the section in Chapter 1 on selecting events to reflect on, to ensure that you maintain a healthy balance in your reflective work.

Selecting your own models and frameworks, or adapting those given to you to suit yourself Part of being successful as a reflective writer is that you are able to select from the array of models and structures available, or even to create your own to suit your particular purpose at the time.

Retaining control over who sees your writing and what they see It is essential that you control the product of the writing. It is up to you to decide who, if anybody, sees your writing – no-one can force you to show what you have written to others. Your first ventures into reflective writing for others may be in classwork, for course assignments or for creating your portfolio. Despite the interpretations often put on these, no-one dictates the content of your writing – you can make choices as to what to use as the subject of your reflective activity, in illustration or evidence that you have achieved the requirements of, for instance, learning outcomes or criteria for the professional body.

> **portfolio**
> A collection of documents that provides evidence of your achievements and professional development

Storing your writing safely Do think about where you will keep your reflective writing once you have done it. Does it need to be in a secret place so that no-one else can access it? Or do you need simply to ensure that it goes into a folder out of the way? If you are writing on computer, does anyone else have access to it, and would it bother you if they read what you had written? One student went as far as only saving his work to a flash drive and storing this in a locked cupboard to prevent others having access to his reflections. You may not have this kind of need for secrecy and security, but giving thought to who might accidentally see your work and planning to avoid this will give you more freedom in what you write and how you write it. Do consider the implications of using social media for your reflective work as well, as often they are not as secure as we would wish. In particular, do ensure that you maintain confidentiality and never identify others by name in your writing.

Planning to complete the reflective cycle The success of writing reflectively, as with any other reflective activity met in this book, is that of completing the reflective cycle. It is often not the subject, or the content, of what you reflect on that is necessarily important, but its analysis in terms of what can be drawn out in understanding and learning. Writing reflectively is simply one way of doing this – one tool in the kit bag – which will suit some people and not others, just as many of the techniques throughout the book will have more appeal to some of us than others.

Over to you

It is clearly up to you who sees your work, and what you choose to do with it. However, these need to be conscious decisions that are taken thoughtfully, if you are to have the safety to write of your own experiences, reactions to them and feelings about them. Developing insight about ourselves is an illuminating and educating process and can bring great satisfaction. It is also risky and can be threatening; therefore we owe it to ourselves to ensure that we minimize risks.

What can you do to ensure that you are safe in your reflective writing?

> ## KEY POINTS
>
> - There are a variety of analytical and creative strategies and styles for reflective writing that can be used to work through the ERA cycle
> - Any of these can be used with a structured framework for reflection
> - It is not, however, necessary to use a structured framework for writing reflectively
> - Writing is a purposive and deliberate activity that helps to provide different insights into our experiences
> - We can take control of our writing and create strategies ourselves for writing safely

Using reflective writing within a portfolio

The aim of this section is to explore ways in which you can incorporate the reflective work that you do within a portfolio. This is intended only as an introduction to the ideas behind portfolio construction and to give you a few pointers to help you.

Both the Health and Care Professions Council and the Nursing and Midwifery Council now ask registered practitioners to keep a record of their continuing professional development as a requirement for periodic registration. Employers are increasingly asking practitioners to present portfolios of their activities over the past year at their annual professional development review and planning session and portfolios are also often required at job interviews. Additionally, portfolios are now recognized as a valuable form of assessment on some courses, and in particular for work-based evidence of achievement of learning outcomes or competencies. In preparation for this, most pre-qualifying health care students are likely to begin starting their portfolios as part of their course. Other students may use portfolios during their course for recording their practice, or as part of coursework. These are usually aimed at enabling the student to recognize their unique and individual development and learning as opposed to the more generic work they do using other forms of assessment.

Hence, the experiences you gain of portfolio work as a student will be preparing you for the professional portfolio you will need to keep once you are qualified. Some of the contents within your portfolio will be your reflective work, which shows how you are applying your knowledge and learning from the experiences you have in practice.

What is a portfolio?

A portfolio is traditionally seen as a collection of documents providing a picture to another person of what the author is like. For instance, an artist might have a portfolio of his work that shows his style and type of work; or a government minister might have a portfolio that outlines her area of responsibility. More recently, the concept of a portfolio has developed within professional practice in terms of documenting and providing evidence of the practitioner's continuing competence and development. This is a movement away from the portfolio as being purely a record of things that have happened to a continuously changing artefact that is used for learning. A definition which brings together the type of portfolios used in health care is provided by Timmins (2008):

> ❝ *A portfolio is ... a cohesive account of work-based learning that contains relevant evidence from practice and critical reflection on this evidence. Its primary purpose is to display achievement of professional competence or learning outcomes and knowledge development.*
>
> *Timmins, 2008, p. 115 in Timmins and Duffy (2011, p. 3)*

Portfolios are used by students in learning contexts to build a collection of evidence. This evidence demonstrates that they are making progress towards achieving the learning outcomes and professional standards expected of them. So the portfolio is constructed for a particular purpose, as opposed to having free content decided by the student. The kinds of document seen in portfolios might include:

- a learning contract
- a list of the learning outcomes to be achieved in the course, module or practice placement
- a list of clinical/practical competencies that need to be achieved
- plans of action for achieving the outcomes and competencies
- reflective reviews of experience
- self-assessment documents
- evidence that demonstrates achievements
- contributions from other people that support the claims being made
- your learning journal or diary
- personal sections in the portfolio that will not necessarily be shown to other people.

Other things that might be included if you are maintaining a general portfolio from which you select specific items for different purposes might be:

- your CV
- your previous job descriptions
- placement descriptions and what you learned within them
- any special skill development
- any achievements or special awards
- your certificates.

You might also want to include material from other people that supports the claims you are making. Examples might be:

- letters that mention your work
- statements from supervisors or others you have worked with
- copies of programmes for study days or conferences you have attended
- reports from clinical practice in which you are mentioned
- evidence that prove that you were a part of something that happened.

This kind of portfolio is essentially a public document because it is being constructed for a specific purpose and is a requirement of a course. There-fore, students need to make decisions about what the portfolio is going to say to the outside world about them, and the kind of picture it will be presenting. It can be compared to compiling a family photograph album. When we choose from all the pictures we have, we want to select those presenting the best possible picture of us. We are unlikely to show others unflattering shots or ones we would be embarrassed about – unless that is specifically what we want to do, of course! So, actively selecting from what we have available to go into the portfolio is very important in creating this picture of ourselves.

Selecting the material for a portfolio

As a student it is likely that a format for the portfolio, and what you are expected to put into it, will be decided for you. But within this, you still have a great deal of leeway in deciding what, from all of your work, will present the best picture of you. Some will be the reflective accounts you have con-structed through the course. Other work to include might be reflections of what you have done independently and want to include because you feel it demonstrates your learning and development.

The ways in which reflective material can be used within the portfolio are:

- in demonstrating achievement of an outcome
- in demonstrating competence
- in academic work to demonstrate learning from experience
- to demonstrate professional development as a practitioner.

When selecting material for the portfolio we need to ask ourselves the following questions:

- What am I using this for?
- What does it say about me as a person?
- What does it say about me as a professional practitioner? How does it demonstrate my learning?
- Can I provide the evidence to show that I have achieved this?

KEY POINTS

- Portfolios are a collection of written material that paint a picture of who we are
- Portfolios are constructed by students for different purposes
- Reflective writing may be used within the portfolio to provide evidence of our achievements

CONCLUSIONS

By necessity this has been a very full and long chapter as we have tried to provide you with concrete ways and examples of how to start 'doing' reflective practice. We hope we have provided you with some practical ways of starting reflective practice by yourself. The illustrations we have used are not meant to be perfect. Rather they are students' own accounts and use of reflective strategies in their own words. Some are beginning students; others are further on in their professional careers. All, though, have effectively used reflective strategies to learn about their practice in some ways. By choosing to use these for yourself, we have no doubt that you too will become a reflective practitioner.

RAPID RECAP

Check your progress so far by working through each of the following questions.

1 What is the difference between reflection-in-action and reflection-on-action?
2 What is reflective writing?
3 What are the features of reflective writing?
4 What are the two categories of reflective writing?
5 How can you plan to write safely?

If you have difficulty with more than one of the questions, read through the section again to refresh your understanding before moving on.

REFERENCES

Allen, D.G., Bowers, B. and Diekelmann, N. (1989) Writing to learn: a reconceptualization of thinking and writing in the nursing curriculum. *Journal of Nursing Education*, 28, 6–11.

Brookfield, S.D. (1987) *Developing Critical Thinkers: Challenging adults to explore alternative ways of thinking and acting.* Jossey Bass, San Francisco.

Facione, P.A., Facione, N.C. and Sanchez, C.A. (1994) Critical thinking disposition as a measure of competent clinical judgment: the development of Critical Thinking Disposition Inven- [ ] *f Nursing Education*, 33, 345–350.

[ ] ngton, A. (2010) *Critical thinking* [ ] *nursing students.* Learning Mat-

[ ] *Making sense of portfolios.* Open [ ] Press, Maidenhead.

Timmins, F. and Duffy, A. (2011) *Writing your nursing portfolio.* RCN publishing company, Maidenhead.

FURTHER READING

My chapters on reflective writing in Rolfe *et al.* 2011, present further examples and illustrations of the ways in which reflective writing can be used by individual practitioners to develop themselves further. Included in this is a useful model of the way that experienced practitioners use reflective writing within their professional portfolios in terms of professional development, personal development, developing critical thinking skills and developing optimal patient care.

Rolfe, G., Freshwater, D. and Jasper, M. (2011) *Critical Reflection in Practice: generating knowledge for care* (2nd edition). Palgrave, Basingstoke.

If you want to understand more about your own writing style, it is worth looking at:

Sharples, M. (1999) *How We Write*, Routledge, London.

Further detail on the use of learning journals in practice-based learning is provided by:

Moon, J. (2006) *Learning journals: a handbook for reflective practice and professional development.* 2nd edition. Routledge, London.

Jasper, M. (2008) 'Using reflective journals and diaries to enhance practice', Chapter 7 in Bulman, C. and Schutz, S. *Reflective Practice in Nursing.* 4th edition. Wiley-Blackwell, Oxford.

You can find further in-depth analysis and strategy for writing reflectively in:

Bolton, G (2010) *Reflective writing and professional development.* 3rd edition. Paul Chapmen Publishing Ltd, London.

CHAPTER 6

WAYS OF REFLECTING WITH OTHERS

LEARNING OBJECTIVES

By the end of this chapter you should be able to:

- identify the benefits of reflecting with others

- explore issues that need careful thinking about before reflecting with others

- identify ways of reflecting with your peers, colleagues and friends

- discuss the use of reflection with clinical mentors, assessors and other professional groups

- explore the use of reflective strategies with educational staff.

In the previous chapter you were encouraged to look at some of the many strategies and ways of reflecting that you can use, whether these be within your professional or personal life. This focused on reflecting by yourself as an individual activity. In this chapter we want you to think about ways to work reflectively with others to enhance your learning opportunities, both formally and informally.

It is inevitable that you start talking about your experiences at university and in clinical placements, and your life in general, with those around you. This will often stray into sharing your successes and triumphs, and musing about problems or things that are worrying you. You may even have had an unpleasant or challenging experience that you are still worrying about; or something has made you angry and you can't get it out of your head. It often helps to be able to mull it over with another person, if only to reassure yourself that what you did was alright.

But, when does simply talking about these things become 'reflective practice'? It is worth reminding ourselves of what we mean by reflective practice as defined in Chapter 1. We identified three components, *experience–reflection–action*, that characterize reflective practice over reflective processes alone. It is the last of these that distinguishes ordinary reflective conversations from actively engaging in reflection with others for the purpose of learning from experience, i.e. the process of identifying action that results in changing practice or resolving a situation. In addition, remember that when doing this in a professional context, both you and the other person have professional responsibilities you need to consider before embarking on conversations which may have consequences for either of you.

So, it is worth thinking about just what it is you are doing and what you want to get out of reflecting with others. Try to think of these as 'formal' processes in order to construct some sort of safety for yourself. Making the decision to reflect with others takes your very personal experiences out of the private domain and into the public one – a cautionary word here is not to take this step lightly! Throughout this book we have encouraged you to make conscious decisions, to choose to reflect and write, to acknowledge that, even in the most mundane of situations, conscious processes are at work, which means that little happens by accident. By actively thinking about our actions and activity, we can acknowledge our own part in this and learn from it. Hence, it is important to think clearly through the issue of reflecting with others so that you do so consciously and with purpose, and with a full understanding of the implications and possible consequences of doing so.

In many ways, it is worth keeping written records of any reflective activity with others, as this serves as a reminder of reflection as a learning process. Similarly, you will be valuing the time spent, and making the most of the activity, if you ensure that you acknowledge this as a strategy for learning. These records can also be a valuable contribution to your course portfolio or learning journal, as they document your development through the course.

THE BENEFITS OF REFLECTING WITH OTHERS

There are many benefits of 'going public' and using reflective strategies with others to help you broaden your views of your experiences. Other people are often better at seeing positive elements of an experience we are finding problematic. This may be because they are more detached and are not caught up in the emotions of what has happened.

Case study

Tom's story – a new student nurse

Tom is an 18-year-old male student nurse, enrolled on the adult field of the BSc (Hons) Nursing programme and is in his second semester of study. He lives at home with his parents and two sisters. He is starting his second practice placement.

"What a day! It was my first day at Sleepwell Nursing Home and I wanted, of course, to make a good impression. There I was in my brand new uniform, with a name badge on and scared stiff of making a fool of myself! I was really glad that Anna, the Clinical Practice Facilitator, had planned to meet me at the home to work with me through the morning. Although I had previously had a ward placement, the environment of a nursing home is very different, not least because the equipment available might not be as up-to-date as that in the NHS. I was to learn this to my cost!

Anna suggested that we build on the skills theory done in class that week, and offered for us to do all the routine observations – temperature, pulse, respirations and blood pressure for all patients. I suppose practice makes perfect, but it seemed a lot, and I thought it would take ages. Practical things aside, as we were talking I realized that there was a lot more about doing observations than just recording the readings. It hadn't occurred to me that the nurse is also observing the patient's general condition, looking for signs of pain and discomfort and assessing their overall mental state through simple conversation.

But, I did learn a lesson that I'll never forget – how could I be so stupid? I was used to using electronic thermometers. The nursing home still used old fashioned mercury thermometers. I had been taught, theoretically, to use these, but because I'd never had to I hadn't really taken in the practical issues involved. The thermometers are all kept in the clinical room and need to be rinsed of the antiseptic solution before use. I felt confident doing this as we talked; I washed, rinsed and dried them, and off we set to the first 'victim'. Anna looked at the first thermometer and suggested I shake it down. Actually, to my embarrassment I couldn't even see the mercury. Anna suggested I try another one, and I couldn't find that either. In fact, I looked at several and none appeared to have any mercury in them. Anna had a wry smile on her face. 'What is the temperature range of these, Tom?' She asked. Then the penny dropped. I'd washed the thermometers in hot soapy water, so every one of them was stuck at the top of the range.

I did feel daft, but having said that, I'll never do it again. I felt a complete idiot, but Anna helped me to see the positive side of it. We had a good giggle actually, and at least the other staff realized that I've got a sense of humour and could laugh at myself. So, although it was a memorable occasion, I really enjoyed the day. The way Anna handled it, and talked it through, turned what could have been humiliating into a positive experience, and also made me realize how important good interpersonal skills are in situations like this. I'll definitely take more notice in 'communications skills' sessions now, even though sometimes the exercises seem a bit obvious. Then again, I didn't think I needed to be told not to wash thermometers in hot water!"

Reflective activity

Consider Tom's story. He has written up his learning journal for his first day on the ward.

- What is the learning that he has identified for himself for the day?
- What has he learned as a result of reflection with Anna?
- What have been the benefits of reflecting with another person here?
- What other benefits may come from reflecting with others?

Some of the things that you might have thought about are:

- Other people can take a more objective stance to something that has happened to you.
- Other people may ask questions that you have not thought of yourself.
- Other people may offer a different way of seeing things.
- Other people can act as a sounding board for your ideas.

- Other people can validate your thoughts about a situation.
- Other people may help you to put events into a different context.
- Other people bring their own knowledge and experiences to the situation, which may help your understanding.
- Other people may offer alternative courses of action to those you have come up with.

Let's explore this a little more.

Taking an objective stance

Emotions often interfere with the way we see things, particularly at the time or when we are still reliving the experience. These emotions are peculiar to you and are wrapped up with both the emotional and physical memories of the experience itself. These memories create your subjective experience. What you remember when retelling the story is not only the words of what happened but also what you were feeling, how you were reacting and the hormonal activity that made up the total experience. This might have included the classic 'fight or flight' reaction, which occurs when you are under stress and causes you to come out of the corner fighting or get tingling feelings, shivers down your back, break out in a sweat, feel sick and want to run away! Another person, even one who was there when the incident took place, will not have the same memories as you, and therefore has a different perspective on what happened. They are more detached simply because they are not you. While another person may be able to empathize with you, they cannot be you, and therefore they are able to be more objective.

We see this in Tom's experience, in that he was so caught up with feeling inadequate at the time that he was unable to rationalize what he was experiencing. It took the objective person to bring his attention back to the incident and focus his thoughts on solving the problem. Anna was able to do this because she was not the one who had had the experience; therefore, she could stand back and concentrate on the problem without having to cope with the emotions and physical reactions that Tom would have been experiencing at the time.

Asking questions that we haven't thought of ourselves

Arising from this objectivity, other people will be able to ask questions you haven't thought of. Some of these will be for clarification, to fill in the gaps you have missed in order to get a complete picture of what happened. These serve the purpose of jogging your memory about the totality of the event, rather than what is uppermost in your mind at the time. In some ways this is similar to the function of using a reflective strategy by yourself – by asking questions through some sort of a framework, you are forced to consider other aspects of the incident that at first may not have seemed so important to you. In a way, this is like finding the corner piece to a jigsaw – your own

Objectivity
Being able to stand back from your own viewpoint and consider all aspects

random thoughts act as the other edge pieces, but the corner piece may be hidden from you and is a key to holding the whole lot together in a coherent structure. While the chances are that you would retrieve these elements for yourself from your memory at some later stage, the other person asking the questions acts as a jolt to your memory.

Reflecting with others can sometimes make
you think of something that completes
the picture and makes sense of it.

Offering a different way of seeing things

Other people also bring their own experience, knowledge and background into the situation, as they in turn reflect on what you are saying. Hence they will be asking questions from their own perspective. Sometimes it is useful to reflect with someone who has a completely different background from you, as different professional groups have differing sets of key theories and will often 'see' a situation through a different set of 'lenses'. For instance, a physiotherapist is likely to understand a person's mobility problems from a different standpoint than that of a nurse or an occupational therapist because of the way they have been taught to use their knowledge base and the perspectives they come from.

Acting as a sounding board for your ideas

Another benefit of using others to reflect with is that they can give immediate feedback to what you are saying. When reflecting by ourselves it is easy to get 'stuck' in a particular train of thought, or to be distracted by your imagination instead of concentrating on exploring the issue at hand. Having another person who will reflect your ideas back to you, or ask for more detail or justification, may help to clarify and validate your own thoughts.

A great benefit of reflecting with others is that they can reinforce your thoughts and actions as reasonable, but also enable you to go beyond what you had been thinking. In terms of reflective practice it is often the other person saying 'Well, what are you going to do about it then?' that spurs us into taking the step from thoughts and ideas to action. Often, if we have told someone else that we are going to do something, it acts as the push to actually doing it – if it remains private and in our own head we always have an excuse for inactivity!

Validating our thoughts about a situation

Often our need to talk about a situation, incident or experience with others stems from an anxiety about what we did or how we are feeling. It is very difficult, unless you are really experienced and skilled at distancing yourself from experiences, to put aside your emotional responses or to validate your own perceptions. In providing a sounding board, another person can act in this capacity. A simple phrase such as 'I would have done that too' or 'That sounds perfectly reasonable to me' will often put our minds at rest, reduce the feelings of discomfort that we have and enable us to see a situation more clearly because the emotional tension has been reduced.

Putting events into a different context

Similarly, another person may be able to go beyond the context of the incident and turn what you saw in a negative light into a positive explanation. The distance this person has may enable them to take a different tack or suggest ways of learning from the situation you haven't been able to think about. Certainly, one of the benefits of clinical supervision is that another practitioner from the same field as yourself can ask questions that force you to think beyond the boundaries you set for yourself and consider or devise strategies for managing situations that may occur.

Bringing alternative knowledge and experience to a situation

Many people we reflect with as students will be experienced practitioners or academic staff who have a wealth of both knowledge and experience to draw on. These people are to be cherished and used for what they can give you! Our understanding of a situation, and the sense we can make of it, relies on the strategies, knowledge and experience that we ourselves have. Other people, however, can call upon different theoretical concepts and their own learning from experience to add to our frameworks. Consider Tom's plight again. He demonstrates a classic example of the theory–practice gap. He draws attention to this himself – if he had been asked if he would wash limited-range thermometers in hot water, he is likely to have laughed and considered the question patronizing. So, if he had stopped to think about what he was doing, he might have acted differently. But he was acting on automatic pilot and had not transformed his knowledge into learning for practice. This illustrates the difference between knowledge and learning – one type of knowledge can be seen as gaining a theoretical understanding about something, whereas learning is related to what you do with the theory and how you use it in the future.

Anna's role, as the teacher, was to help Tom make the connections between his actions and the theory underpinning them. This is not to say Tom would not have reached the same conclusions by himself. Using Anna was a shortcut to something he would have achieved alone at a later date (or even in the next few minutes!). Anna's knowledge came from a combination of theory in action and experience of being in the situation many times before. She was able to determine the cause of the problem before Tom as a result of familiarity with a situation she had met previously. She had even possibly had experience with another student doing just the same as Tom! Her experience as a teacher, however, also led her to believe that we learn as a result of doing something – hence, rather than reminding Tom to use tepid water to rinse the thermometers, she allowed him to go ahead and then to learn from his error. This is 'discovery' learning, and is often a far more powerful source of learning (or behaviour change) than doing things because we are told to and don't have the opportunity to test out alternatives for ourselves.

Offering alternative courses of action

Finally, because of their distance from the experience, other people may offer alternative courses of action, beyond those we can see ourselves. This is particularly important in professional contexts, as experienced mentors have a repertoire of paradigm cases to draw from that enable them to chose from a number of different courses of action, even though the situation they are dealing with appears the same. This enables us to take account of individuality and treat people according to their own particular circumstances, rather than applying blanket patterns of care to all. A good reflective facilitator will enable us to expand our own horizons using reflective techniques, so we draw our own conclusions about the appropriateness of certain courses of action, resulting in empowerment and taking control.

Case study

Heidi's story

Heidi is a 20-year-old physiotherapy student who has started her third year of study.

"I know that Ben has a lot of experience, and that I could learn a lot from him, but he really seems to be down on me the whole time; I don't think he likes me at all. Take today for instance. Mrs Jones is really hard to motivate to mobilize, but she won't be able to go home until she can get in and out of bed by herself, go to the bathroom, move from her chair to the kitchen, and other things that she needs to get around her flat. Ben and I were going to the ward to help her do some exercises and reassess her progress and plans when Ben, all of a sudden, just said: 'You take the lead on this one'. Well, I had visited her by myself before a couple of times, as well as with Ben, but this came as a bit of a shock. I'm used to planning interventions and really thinking about what I'm trying to achieve with a patient before I go to see them. I thought as Ben was there that he was taking the lead, especially as this was a review visit.

So, I was totally unprepared really. That, and Ben being there, made me really nervous. I must have seemed a complete idiot to Mrs Jones, and usually we get on really well. I forgot loads of things on the assessment, and I could tell that Ben was getting more and more irritated with me. Things got worse when we were trying to help Mrs Jones walk alone down the ward using her frame; each thought the other was supporting her. When she stumbled, neither of us was correctly positioned to steady her and she ended up on the floor. That meant that an incident form had to be filled out, and we had to use the hoist to get her back up off the ground. She was really upset, had a big bruise on her hip and was very shaken. This meant that we had to abandon trying any more work with her, and spent the time reassuring her.

Ben was really angry afterwards, and said it was all my fault. He completely ignored me when he fed back to the nurses on duty, updated her schedule without consulting me or asking me what I thought, and stormed off, leaving me to trot behind like a little puppy."

Reflective activity

Take some time now to think about the benefits of reflecting with other people.

Consider Heidi's dilemma as she recorded it in her reflective diary.

Imagine that you are Heidi's flatmate, and also a health care student but from a different discipline. List the questions that you would use if she came home after this incident and wanted to talk about it.

First, how could you help her to learn from what has happened so that she can:

- talk to Ben about what happened with Mrs Jones
- identify ways of working with Ben for the future
- manage her own reactions to unplanned situations
- develop assertive behavioural strategies and communication for dealing with similar situations again
- decide whether she needs to talk to anyone else more formally about this, perhaps her personal tutor at the University.

Second, think about the benefits of reflecting with others. How many of these would have applied to your talk with Heidi?

Third, what might be some of the pitfalls of reflecting with other people, and how could you plan to avoid these occurring?

ISSUES TO THINK ABOUT BEFORE STARTING A REFLECTIVE RELATIONSHIP WITH ANOTHER PERSON

While reflecting with others can be an enriching and enlightening experience, there are issues it is worth considering before doing so. Some of the reflective work you do with other people will be in an informal setting, such as with your friends, colleagues and peers or at home with your partner or relatives. These opportunities will be under your control and often at your discretion – you can choose to start conversations with others, seek them out and perhaps affect the direction in which things go. However, as a student, it is likely that you will have reflective situations imposed upon you; and you may not have much choice about strategies for reflecting with others during your course. Such strategies in educational settings might be:

- reflective group work with your peers
- one-to-one tutorials with a lecturer or tutor
- clinical supervision with your mentor/assessor
- using written reflective work in seminars
- role play using reflective strategies
- written reflective reviews and work for your portfolio that will be seen by others either informally or for assessment purposes.

In each of these, do remember that you are able to make decisions about what part you play in these activities and how much of your personal work, or yourself, you disclose. No one can force you to give personal information, or discuss experiences that may be uncomfortable for you, in a public arena. This includes tutorials with your lecturers. Similarly, even if some form of reflective writing, such as a learning journal, reflective review or diary, is compulsory, you can choose what other people see and what you submit for assessment.

Remember also that reflection with others is seen as a strategy for learning – any situation in which you do this will be considered as a formal occasion, no matter how informal the setting, the environment or the atmosphere. Hence, it is worth approaching reflection with others having considered the issues and established some parameters for yourself.

Over to you

Remind yourself of what you wrote for the final part of the previous task. Do you want to add any more to it before reading further?

Establishing the purpose of the encounter

You will find yourself in reflective encounters that take many different forms. However, to get the most out of them try to spend a few minutes thinking about what you want to achieve as a result of it, and planning to make sure this happens.

*Reflect**Reflective activity***

Why do you do what you do?

Look back at your answers to Heidi's problem. Clearly, this situation arose spontaneously and you would have responded as a friend or colleague rather than in any planned or formal written way. But can you think of how you might have handled the situation differently if you had been able to think about the encounter in advance? If you had been able to negotiate outcomes with Heidi, what might these have been?

When you are with friends, or even in a working relationship, it is easy to slip into talking over events and things that have happened. You'll probably be more aware of this at the outset of any reflective activity you have with your mentor/supervisor and your educational advisors. Encounters with the last two groups are likely to be more formal, planned and focused on outcomes that are predefined. These may be about identifying your learning as a result of work you have done in placement, and end up in defining what more you need to achieve, or follow up on. They might also be about your progress so far, how you are doing against set criteria for the placement, and planning for the rest of your time there. Yet another type of reflective event may be specifically about an incident that has happened, where you spend time exploring what has occurred, to learn from it and for it to become one of your own paradigm cases.

Similarly, in an educational setting, the chances are that lecturers will focus on what they want you to achieve as a result of the reflective work. But this doesn't stop you thinking about it beforehand and planning your own objectives and outcomes. This is particularly so if you have a one-to-one tutorial that has a time limit and there are specific things you want to know about or achieve. Lecturers are usually busy people and need to make the most of tutorial time. They will appreciate you spending a little time thinking through what you want from the tutorial and coming along armed with a list, and pen and paper to make notes as you go along. This can be especially important if you are asking for advice on assignments coming up you have queries about. It is easy to sit and think 'I'll remember that' and then get outside and realize you haven't taken in a word that was said! It is also worth writing up your tutorials and using them as a focus for reflection, in terms of capitalizing on your learning from others and the communication strategies you develop in negotiating with educational staff.

All three types of encounter will have more benefit if you plan what it is you want out of them before you start. This needn't take long, but setting a few goals to focus your mind and planning to achieve outcomes makes the most effective use of your time, and the other person's. Similarly, writing up the event in your learning journal provides you with the time to think things over and create a record. In particular, getting into the habit of concisely identifying what you feel you have learned each day provides an on-going record of your progress and development.

So, here are a few useful tips to think about before embarking on reflective sessions with someone else:

- Establish the purpose of the encounter with the other person at the outset.
- Be aware of what you are saying and the implications that this might have.
- Think about setting boundaries/rules of engagement/outcomes.
- Be prepared to accept that others may have different views from you and that these are not only valid but worthy of consideration.
- Be aware of what you are asking the other person to do – either as the person reflecting on an experience or as another person in the reflective relationship.
- Take a few minutes after the encounter to summarize the main points for yourself and plan any action.

The nature of the relationship

The nature of the relationship you have with the person will have an effect on several aspects of the event. The types of people you will be working with fall into three main groups:

- friends, peers, colleagues, partners and family
- professional workers – your mentor/supervisor or assessor, other workers in your own discipline and members of other professions
- educational staff – your lecturers, link tutors in clinical placements, your personal tutor, etc.

Clearly, you will have a different sort of relationship with the people in each of these groups, and this will affect the type of reflective work you do with them. Three issues are of particular importance here.

Issues of trust

Being able to trust the people you reflect with is of crucial importance if you are going to learn from the work you do. This can take many forms. First of all, you need to feel comfortable with the person, whether that means you appear to be on the same wavelength, that you talk the 'same language', that you feel they will not be judgemental or that they allow you the space to talk without interrupting. Secondly, you need to have faith in the other person's judgement; consider whether you think they can offer sound advice that is in your best interests and whether they have the information, knowledge and experience you need. Finally, perhaps you need to consider the other person's interpersonal skills and how they communicate with you. Do they truly listen and empathize with you and are they able to reflect back to you in a caring way, helping you come to a different understanding of your situation?

Confidentiality

Another way in which we need to be able to trust people we reflect with is to be reassured that the conversation is private and that elements of it will not be spread around to others. This is a difficult issue, because very often we do not think we need to say 'This is just between you and me' or 'I would not want anyone else to know about this'. This is especially so when it is our friends that we are talking with and we take it as read that we can trust them in this way.

However, the boundaries are not so clear when it comes to reflecting in a professional capacity, as your mentor or tutor may feel that the issue is of wider concern and they need to consult with other people. Take Heidi's experience, for instance. As a result of your talk with her, she might have decided to go to her tutor at university and talk about her problem. In turn, the tutor may decide s/he needs to intervene in the student/mentor relationship, as there are clearly problems here that need resolving if Heidi is to have a successful learning experience under Ben's mentorship.

The implications here are that clear boundaries need to be set from the beginning of any reflective activity with other people. If, at the start of a conversation you clearly state that what you are going to say is of a delicate nature and at this time you do not want it to go any further than the people in the room, then they have the opportunity to say whether or not they can abide by that. It is up to them to say if they can keep to your rules. If they have reservations and feel they may need to take something further, then you also have the option of not sharing with them what you were going to say, and seeking out a different forum. Similarly, of course, if you are the one listening, you need to consider your own commitment to confidentiality, and whether you are able to keep other people's confidences to yourself. Some people find it difficult to keep secrets or, may inadvertently act on information that has been received in confidence. If you know your best friend, or the tutor you talk to, has a tendency to do this, you have the choice of talking to them or not. If you know you find it difficult not to use information, or to keep a confidence, it is only fair to the person talking to you to say this and allow them to make the decision about whether or not to carry on.

The issue of confidentiality also arises when talking, or writing, about other people, in particular where patients and clients are involved, or other ward staff. As a student in a professional capacity, you have a responsibility to respect the confidentiality of others and not to make information about them public. So, if you are planning to use your experiences with patients as the basis for reflective work, do ensure that anything you use is anonymous and is not likely to identify the person concerned. In particular, it is important to consider your use of social media, such as Facebook and Twitter, very, very carefully before using them as media for your reflective work, or indeed, any postings about clients or people you work with at all.

Case study

Hanif loses his cool

Hanif is a 25-year-old student in his second, and final, year of study on the Diploma of Paramedic Studies. He has received a letter from his programme leader telling him that he is facing serious disciplinary charges, which might result in his being removed from the programme as a result of a posting he made on Facebook. This referred to both his practice mentor and a patient by name. He used Borton's framework to reflect on the incident.

What happened? "I had a really bad day on Monday last week, Rashid (my paramedic mentor) and I went to a filthy sixth floor flat in the Ratmouth estate answering an emergency call that sounded like domestic abuse. Rashid warned me beforehand to be very careful about my own safety as well as ensuring we stuck strictly to our roles as paramedics and did not become involved in whatever was going on. We found a severely beaten woman, and two terrified children in the house, A very drunk man was being restrained by the police, and was taken away in a police car. We stabilized the woman, calmed the children down before social workers arrived to arrange for them to be looked after by their Aunt, and transferred the woman to hospital. I was so upset by what I saw – I don't understand how men can beat women up like this, that I poured it all out on my Facebook page, including names of people involved and places. Someone read the page and reported me to the University."

So what? "Even though I'm not yet registered, as a paramedic I am expected to conduct myself, at all times, according to the guidance provided by the HPC (2009) and respect the confidentiality of my service users. Also I should not do anything to bring my profession into disrepute. I knew all of this, but the incident was just so frustrating, I was shocked at my first 'domestic' and just poured it all out on Facebook. I know I shouldn't have done it, and took it down as soon as I'd thought about it, but, the harm had already been done."

Now what? "I know the University is very strict about poor professional behaviour. At least this isn't a criminal charge that will result in me having a police record. I can only hope that I will get a warning about this incident and that no further action will be taken. I know it is serious though, and risk being removed from the programme. I will never, ever, use Facebook to record anything to do with work again."

Over to you

Hanif's experience is not unusual. It is very easy to use writing on social media as a reaction to things that have happened to us and as an outlet. However, as student professional practitioners, you need to be aware that your behaviour at any time, if it contravenes your professional code of conduct, may have serious implications for your qualification and your registration. Take some time to consider how you currently use social media of any kind, and assess whether you are putting yourself at risk.

Assessment

Many of the people you reflect with will also be acting as your assessors in some way. This includes people who will formally assess you by marking your work or completing your practical assessment documents, those that you work with and other lecturers, who will be feeding in to your overall course assessment. Anyone who is responsible for assessing you has a dual role. Not only will they be guiding and teaching you throughout the time you are with them but they will also be making judgements about you, your learning and your competence to practise. At the end of the day, it is your assessors who approve your licence to practise; it is their judgement that determines whether you will qualify as a professional practitioner or not. This means that sometimes it is worth being cautious about who you choose to reflect with, and what it is you disclose.

Identifying the nature of the relationship you have with the people you choose to reflect with is important in planning for your reflective activity to be successful. Remember, everyone is not there to be your friend – they all have their own professional roles and responsibilities in interacting with you, and this will determine the kind of the interaction you have with them. Acknowledging this and planning to use it in a positive way is crucial in ensuring you enter a reflective relationship feeling secure and being able to trust that person. Thinking about this in advance and planning the interaction to come will help you to feel you have some control, as will negotiating the boundaries for the interaction and the ground rules under which it continues.

Setting boundaries and ground rules for reflecting with others

This sounds a rather formal and intimidating step to take. In reality, once you get used to doing this it not only ensures that both you and the other person have a clear understanding of what it is you are there to do, it also helps you to use your time effectively and achieve what you want from the encounter.

Time and place

There are some basic elements that might sound obvious. First of all, think about what kind of environment and setting you will feel happiest and most relaxed in. Being clear about the time you are going to meet, the amount of time you will spend reflecting with the other person and where you will do this, clearly establishes the activity as a formal appointment with some purpose. It will signal a commitment from both of you and acknowledge that there is serious work to be done – you are not just turning up for a chat!

Choosing a place to work in has a dramatic effect on how relaxed you will feel, how secure and safe you will be and to what extent you are able to settle into a conversation. A review of your progress with your assessor, for instance, is not likely to be confidential if it is carried out in an office with open access to other people, phones ringing and others working at desks. You are unlikely to feel confident discussing issues you feel should be kept between the two of you in this sort of environment. Developing assertive skills, by suggesting a more appropriate environment prior to the meeting, avoids any problems of this sort on the day.

You should always insist on a suitable setting
for your reflective meetings.

The focus of the meeting

Again, if the focus of the meeting is negotiated in advance it allows both sides in the encounter the chance to plan and gather information. This might simply be that you ensure you have notes about the issue before you attend the meeting, and that you have already reflected by yourself on what it is that you want to achieve by the end. It also gives the other person an idea of what the issue or issues may be and they can ensure that they have the relevant information, documentation, etc. so the most is made of the time available.

The other person may have initiated the meeting and have their own agenda – again, if you can have a part in this it enables you to feel that you have some control in the encounter and you are valued as an equal in the process. For instance, if you have booked a tutorial to talk about a draft assignment, it is important that you have submitted it in good time to allow your tutor to have read it and make comments. Turning up with the assignment in your hand is unfair – your tutor cannot give you adequate feedback while reading the work in front of you. However, if you have let them have it in advance, it is reasonable on your part to assume that they will have read it and will be able to use the time effectively in feedback. Equally, it is unfair for another person to ask you to see them without letting you know what the meeting is about – we must all have experienced the call to the headteacher's office at school as a child. Past experiences of this sort can influence how we approach meetings in the future. Always try to go back to a person and establish the topic of the meeting to enable you to prepare for it in advance – this helps both parties, as you will have collected any significant information, and are more likely to be relaxed during the interaction.

Identifying the meeting's outcomes

Managing the content and focus of reflective meetings in this way ensures that you focus on the issue identified and that you are setting up the meeting to be effective. The next thing to think about is what it is that you want to achieve as a result of the meeting.

One of the most satisfying aspects of reflecting with other people is that you can plan to find answers, solutions and prescribe action as a result of the encounter, when you might not be able to do so by yourself. Some meetings will have easily definable outcomes, such as identifying further library work needed in order to understand the theory behind something you have encountered in practice. At other times, however, it is not so simple. Often, we go into reflective activities with others without having envisaged a tangible outcome. We might think things like 'I just want to know what to do' or 'I want to get this sorted out'. This is, in fact a good place to start. Turning these into outcomes you can phrase in an objective way starts the reflective process and enables you to begin stepping back from the situation and creating a distance between you and the event. If it is possible to do this before the meeting, and go into it with clearly defined objectives, then you have already done a lot of the work.

However, it is not essential to do this; what is essential is that you start off the meeting by exploring with the other person what you, and they, want to achieve.

Managing the meeting

You also have to consider, however, how the meeting will work. Ground rules for the meeting itself, and the parts people play within it, bear some thinking about. When there are only two of you, it may be important that the balance of the conversation is skewed in one direction, depending on the meeting's focus and intention. Issues that you might like to consider are:

- how both people will be able to say what they want to say in safety
- the type of language that you will use
- how you will manage confidentiality
- what role you will each play in the meeting
- how you determine the action that both people will take as a result of the meeting
- how you will record the meeting.

This probably all sounds very complicated, and you may be wondering if it is all worth it. Not all meetings you have will work like this. You will not be in the position of being able to think through these processes and get everything sorted out in your mind every time you plan to meet up with another person for reflective activity. But, equally, there will be occasions where you are able to do this, and it is worth taking five minutes or so beforehand to ensure you make the most effective use of your time with the other person. Taking responsibility for your own learning is the key to reflective practice. A conscious use of the processes of learning from reflection will enable you to achieve your outcomes more quickly and effectively than simply waiting for things to happen.

KEY POINTS

- Choose the time and place to suit the type of encounter, and keep to them.
- Identify the focus of the meeting and negotiate what both parties will do in preparation for it.
- Write down what you want to achieve from the meeting and negotiate with the other person what they want to get out of it.
- Talk about confidentiality at the start of the meeting if this is appropriate.
- Agree ground rules about the way the meeting is conducted.

Considering the risks of reflecting with others

What does this mean? In any encounter with another person there will be risks involved. When using reflection as a tool to learn from experience, there is always a range of outcomes that may occur because the subject of the reflection is, in the majority of cases, something that has happened to you, which means you have an emotional stake in the experience. Although the focus of any reflective activity can come from the whole range of your experiences, often it is those that have left you feeling uncomfortable, or where you are unhappy with the outcome, that are the subject of your reflective activity. These, then, also have the potential to cause us more stress because they have arisen from situations in which we have felt vulnerable and out of control. For instance:

- you might not like what others say to you
- you might feel uncomfortable with the 'reflective mirror' others hold up to you
- you may feel overpowered or taken in directions that you do not feel comfortable with
- you may feel others are judging you
- you may feel you are under attack
- you may feel you have done something wrong
- you may feel you lack control in the encounter.

Anticipating the risks of a reflective encounter helps prepare you for what you may experience. Probably the most important way of doing this is to use the stages of the process outlined in the previous sections to move your perception of the meeting from focusing on something you have done to a chance to learn from experience. Creating a distance from the focus of the encounter helps us to use the experience of others to maximum effect. In particular, negotiating ground rules for conducting the meeting is vital to avoid situations such as those described above; learning is unlikely to occur if you feel threatened and attacked by what happens during the meeting.

KEY POINTS

- Use the ground rules previously negotiated to keep the conduct of the meeting fair and equitable to all.
- Use the meeting's facilitator (in a group situation) if you feel under threat.
- Be clear in stating to the group/other person if you feel unhappy about what is happening.
- Focus on the outcomes you want to achieve.
- Never ask a question you don't really want an answer to, or if you haven't prepared yourself for an answer you weren't expecting.
- Try to end the encounter on a positive note.

The professional and/or ethical implications

All health care professionals work within professional codes of conduct and ethics (HPC, 2004, NMC, 2008), whether formal or informal. An example of a code of principles is that of the Nursing and Midwifery Council (2008), which states:

> The people in your care must be able to trust you with their health and wellbeing.
> To justify this you must:
>
> - Make the care of people your first concern, treating them as individuals and respecting their dignity
> - Work with others to protect and promote the health and wellbeing of those in your care, their families and carers, and the wider community
> - Provide a high standard of practice and care at all times
> - Be open and honest, act with integrity and uphold the reputation of your profession.
>
> As a professional, you are personally accountable for actions and omissions in your practice, and must always be able to justify your decisions.
> You must always act lawfully, whether those laws relate to your professional practice or your personal life.
> Failure to comply with this code may bring your fitness to practise into question and endanger your registration.
>
> *Nursing and Midwifery Council (2008, p. 2),*
> *available at* **www.nmc-uk.org**

Each of these four duties are explained in further detail, in terms of how the practitioner can demonstrate they practise to the prescribed standard.

Similarly, the Health Professions Council leaves its registrants in no doubt as to their responsibilities as registrants in their Standards of conduct, performance and ethics (2004, pp. 4–5) as shown below.

> As a health professional, you must protect the health and wellbeing of people who use or need your services in every circumstance. This means that you must always keep high standards of conduct. You must always:
>
> 1 Act in the best interests of your patients, clients and users;
> 2 Respect the confidentiality of your patients, clients and users;
> 3 Maintain high standards of personal conduct; and
> 4 Provide any important information about conduct, competence or health. Also, you must always keep high standards of performance. You must always

  5 *Keep your professional knowledge and skills up to date;*

  6 *Act within the limits of your knowledge, skills and experience and, if necessary, refer on to another professional;*

  7 *Maintain proper and effective communications with patients, clients, users, carers and professionals;*

  8 *Effectively supervise tasks you have asked others to carry out for you;*

  9 *Get informed consent to give treatment (except in an emergency);*

 10 *Keep accurate patient, client and user records;*

 11 *Deal fairly and safely with the risks of infection; and*

 12 *Limit your work or stop practising if your performance or judgement is affected by your health.*

Finally, you must always keep high standards of ethics. You must always:

 13 *Carry out your duties in a professional and ethical way;*

 14 *Behave with integrity and honesty;*

 15 *Follow our guidelines for how to advertise your services; and*

 16 *Make sure that your behaviour does not damage your profession's reputation.*

The Health and Care Professions Council (formed in 2003 and known until September 2012 as the Health Professions Council), brings together the previously separate professions allied to medicine, social care and social work for registration and regulatory purposes. Part of its area of responsibility is to ensure that all professions within their remit work within an established code of conduct incorporating standards for practice and ethical guidelines.

Therefore, it is important to remember that, whenever you are reflecting with other people in a professional capacity (even with other students), you must be aware of the responsibilities that you and the other person have according to the code of conduct. Many of the events you reflect upon and use as the focus for reflective encounters with other people will be incidents that have caused you to be uncomfortable in some way. These might involve what you consider to be unsatisfactory standards of care given to patients or clients; misconduct or negligence by another member of staff; abuse of patients, particularly vulnerable people such as children, the elderly or people with learning disabilities; or episodes of care you find ethically suspect.

Case study

Jim is an unwilling witness

Jim is a third year Speech and Language Therapy student, aged 24 years, and starting to take responsibility for some aspects of practice independently.

Jim was working with Mrs W on Buttercup Ward, assessing her swallowing after she had had a stroke. He became aware of raised voices in the single room next door and couldn't help hearing what was going on. The nurse was trying to change the dressings on Mr T's legs. This was not an easy or pleasant task for either of them because his leg ulcers were extensive and had an unpleasant-smelling exudate that dried between dressings, making them very difficult to remove. Mr T hated having his dressings done because it was very painful. The nurses gave him painkillers before the procedure, and offered him gas and air during the worst bits.

On this occasion though it was obvious that things weren't going right. Mr T was telling the nurse she wasn't doing it right, and to leave him alone. The nurse seemed to lose her temper, called him an ungrateful old man and said that she was going to do what she had to. She then gave him a few home truths, which, as an unwilling witness, Jim found embarrassing. He wasn't sure what happened next, but he heard what sounded like someone being slapped. Mr T grunted and it all went very quiet. A few minutes later the nurse came out of the room, and Jim looked in to see if Mr T was all right. He noticed what looked like a fresh bruise on Mr T's face.

Reflective activity

What should Jim do next?

Imagine you were the one who witnessed this happening, and decided to use it as the focus for a reflective tutorial with your tutor.

- What would you want to achieve from the tutorial?
- What are the implications within your professional code of conduct in terms of:
  - Your responsibility towards the patient concerned
  - Your responsibility towards the nurse
  - Your professional responsibility as a student practitioner in maintaining standards and ensuring patient safety
  - Confidentiality?
- What responsibility did Jim's supervisor have on hearing the story?
- What might be the implications for the tutor you are discussing it with?

In sharing issues of this kind with other people, you must be aware that action might need to be taken as a result of what you have said. This can be extremely difficult for all concerned, and it is vital you consider these issues before deciding to talk to others about incidents with an element of professional misconduct. Other registered practitioners have a duty, as do you, to report any incident where standards of care and the professional code of conduct are breached.

You may not have witnessed such an incident but may actually have done something that contravenes the code of conduct yourself. We need to bear the code of professional conduct in mind all the time and attempt to achieve professionally acceptable standards of behaviour in everything we do. This includes:

- The ways in which we speak to and of other people
- The type of language we use with others
- The ways in which we act in the clinical environment, including how we touch others
- The ways in which we treat other people
- The consideration we give to respecting others and maintaining their dignity
- Attempting to do our patients and clients no harm
- Acting in the patients' best interests
- The impression we give others when we are not in the clinical environment, e.g. the message others may get if they see a nurse smoking when in uniform as well as the more clinical or practical elements of our job.

KEY POINTS

When considering reflecting with others in a professional context, think about:

- the contextual implications of discussing things that have happened
- choosing what to tell and considering the implications of this
- working within professional codes of conduct and discuss the implications of this
- the consequences of disclosure
- misconduct/malpractice/negligence
- understanding the responsibilities of others within their professional role.

CONTEXTS FOR REFLECTING WITH OTHERS

Finally, we need to think about the context in which we reflect with other people. First of all, the issues to be considered when you are engaging in reflective work with one other person, and when you will be part of a group using reflective techniques for learning. Secondly we want to look at the differing issues involved when you are reflecting with the three groups of people who have a part in your education.

Reflecting in a one-to-one relationship

There are two primary relationships that occur when you are reflecting with one other person. First, there is the informal relationship you have with your peers, colleagues, fellow students, friends and relatives. Second, there is the more formal type of relationship you have with your supervisor, other professional colleagues and your academic tutors.

The nature of the relationship you have with members of each of these groups is, by necessity, different – the only reason you have a relationship with the second group is because you are a student.

Reflective activity

Reflecting on a one-to-one basis has certain benefits:

- What might these benefits be?
- What might the disadvantages be?

In preparing for any reflective activity with another person in a one-to-one relationship, we can summarize the issues as:

- setting ground rules and boundaries; contracts
- establishing purposes and outcomes
- defining responsibilities
- framing action.

Reflecting in a group

You are likely to find yourself reflecting as a group within two main contexts. Most probably, you will use group work in an educational setting, facilitated by a lecturer or practitioner. However, you may also find yourself in a group in the practice environment, as more and more clinical areas establish reflective practice techniques in the workplace for continual professional development. Some areas may do this specifically for all the students in their specialty.

Reflecting in a group is an extremely valuable way of broadening your perspective on an issue, as you will meet with others whose views are not known to you and who can bring entirely different experiences into the group. However, while working reflectively in groups has benefits, again, there are issues about the dynamics of groups, and the risks inherent in several people being involved, needing to be thought through.

Reflect*Reflective activity*

What will be different about reflecting in a group from reflecting with just one person? How can you plan to use these features effectively to maximize your learning?

Some of the issues you may have thought about are:

- Who is facilitating the group, and what are their roles and responsibilities
- Establishing the ground rules and boundaries for the life of the group
- Establishing the commitment of the group members
- Ensuring you feel safe – this relates to what you are prepared to say in the group setting and who you are prepared to say it to
- Agreeing rules for confidentiality
- Identifying the purpose of the group
- Identifying the learning that has been achieved
- Framing action as a result on both a group and personal basis.

Reflecting with peers, colleagues and friends

When you can choose the person you talk to, maybe a friend, another student or a member of your family, you have a large element of control within the encounter and are likely to feel safer and more secure in the way you talk to them. With these people you have a complex set of relationships that change with the different roles you are in. These informal relationships enable you to take a very different approach to reflection with another person from when you are in a working relationship with them. As a result, the reflecting you do is likely to be less formal and less structured. You may find that you rarely use a framework for reflection with these people, unless you specifically set out to do so.

Reflect*Reflective activity*

- What might be the advantages of reflecting with someone with whom you have a friendship, relationship, or informal acquaintance?
- What might the drawbacks be?
- How can you use these to reflect effectively with this group of people?

Using mentors/assessors and clinical supervision

Similarly, reflecting with this group of people will have its own character. These people are not only in a professional relationship with you and have certain responsibilities towards you in that capacity, they are also members of a profession themselves and therefore act as gatekeepers for that profession. Hence, the reflective work you do with them will be more formal in its nature, and probably directed at achieving specific purposes.

Reflective activity

Think again about the benefits these features bring to the reflective encounters.
What issues will you need to think about before this type of activity?

These last two activities are really asking you to review what you have learned from the previous sections of this chapter and apply it to yourself.

The contexts in which you may be reflecting with this group of people are:

- Establishing your learning needs at the beginning of a placement
- Clinical supervision/formal reflective sessions throughout the placement
- Reflective reviews of your learning
- **Tripartite** meetings with your practice supervisor/mentor and link teacher or academic advisor
- Informal reflective sessions
- To take action (reflecting)
- Talking after the action (reflection on action)
- Seeking others out in response to things that have happened
- Sharing ideas

Tripartite
Involving three
people

Using academic staff

Finally, we turn to your relationship with the academic staff. Again, this relationship has a different nature and context from those involving the other groups of people.

Reflective activity

- What are the special features of your relationship with academic staff?
- How do these differ from those you have with others?
- How can you plan to use these features in working reflectively with academic staff?

All the academic staff you work with will have several functions within their relationship with you. Some of these are:

- as a teacher
- as a facilitator
- as a personal tutor
- as a confidante
- as a clinical tutor/link lecturer
- as a marker/assessor of your work and progress
- as a professional gatekeeper
- as a maintainer of standards
- as a supporter.

Their primary role may be to support you in your learning throughout your course. But they also have professional responsibilities belonging to their roles as an employee of an academic institution and as a member of their profession. These two roles both carry a responsibility for upholding standards, and this is bound up within the relationship they have with you. As a result, any reflective work you do with them will be framed within these three functions.

Reflective activity

In this last activity, we want you to think about the types of reflective encounter that you might have with academic staff. Use the list of the lecturer's functions above as a focus.

- What might you want to achieve from these?
- How can you plan to use these to your advantage?

Within all these contexts, each person in the relationship has their own agenda and responsibilities. Your primary role as a student will ensure that you are using the reflective processes involved to learn and develop towards being a professional practitioner. While these will certainly be a part of the intentions of the others involved, they will also have different purposes for the activities. Therefore, it is up to you to think about each encounter in advance and plan to achieve what it is you need. This may even involve taking some sort of control during the meeting to ensure your needs are met as well as the other person's. It always helps if you plan in advance, and maybe even go along with a list of the things you want to achieve as a guide for the time you have available. This will help you to make the most of this and ensures you maximize your learning.

KEY POINTS

- We can use the different relationships we have with others for different kinds of reflection.
- One-to-one reflection has a different nature from group reflection.
- Forward planning before any reflective encounter with others will ensure our own needs are met.
- Remember that every person involved in a reflective relationship has differing needs from it and will be working to achieve these.
- The primary responsibility for the student's learning within reflective encounters lies with the student.

CONCLUSIONS

Throughout this chapter we have tried to take a balanced view of the advantages and challenges of reflecting with other people. This is clearly different from reflecting by yourself. While it brings huge rewards in helping you to see different perspectives and think about your experiences in different ways, it also carries certain risks and vulnerabilities with it that need active management and forward planning.

As with all reflective activity, the more you think about what you want to achieve by reflecting with other people, the more you are likely to get from it. By identifying the learning outcomes so that you are able to take some sort of action, you will be completing the ERA cycle every time. As a result, you will be functioning as a reflective practitioner in all the contexts in which you operate.

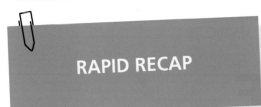

RAPID RECAP

Check your progress so far by working through each of the following questions.

1 What are the benefits of reflecting with others?

2 What different groups of people could you choose to reflect with?

3 What issues do you need to think about before starting to reflect with others?

4 How can you make the most of reflecting with others?

If you have difficulty with more than one of the questions, read through the section again to refresh your understanding before moving on.

REFERENCES

Nursing and Midwifery Council (2008) *The code: Standards of conduct, performance and ethics for nurses and midwives*. NMC, London. **www.nmc-uk.org**.

Health Professions Council (2004) *Standards of conduct, performance and ethics*. HPC, London, **www.hpc-uk.org**

FURTHER READING

We have not gone into a lot of detail about clinical supervision here, but this is clearly an area where reflective practice is encouraged and developed. The following sources will provide you with further understanding of it.

Bond, M. and Holland, S. (2011) *Skills of Clinical Supervision for Nurses: a practical guide for supervisees* (2nd edition). OUP, Maidenhead, UK.

Bulman, C. and Schutz, S. (2008) *Reflective practice in nursing* (4th edition). Blackwell Publishing, Oxford.

Contains a chapter on group reflection by Bernie Carter and Elizabeth Walker.

Rolfe, G., Freshwater, D. and Jasper, M. (2011) *Critical Reflection in practice: generating knowledge for care* (2nd edition). Palgrave, Basingstoke.

This book has two chapters about clinical supervision, which provide a useful outline of the principles of both individual and group supervision.

MAPPING OF CHAPTERS TO NMC STANDARDS AND ESSENTIAL SKILLS CLUSTERS

Chapter number, title and learning outcomes	NMC Standards for Pre-registration Nursing Education (2010)		Essential skills cluster	
	Domain	Competency	Cluster	Skill
1: What is reflective practice? Understand the concept of reflective practice Distinguish between reflective processes and reflective practice Appreciate how reflection can be seen as a strategy for learning Understand how learning can occur from experience and recognize opportunities for learning within a working environment Understand how reflective practice can help to bridge theory and practice.	Professional Values	**1.1** All nurses must practice with confidence according to The Code: Standards of Conduct, performance and Ethics for nurses and midwives (NMC 2008) and within other recognized ethical and legal frameworks. **1.7** All nurses must be responsible and accountable for keeping their knowledge and skills up to date through continuing professional development. They must aim to improve their performance and enhance the safety of care through evaluation, supervision and appraisal. **1.8** All nurses must practice independently, recognizing the limits of their competence and knowledge. They must **reflect** on these limits and seek advice from, or refer to, other professionals where necessary.	**Care, Compassion and Communication**	**1.** As partners in the care process, people can trust a newly registered graduate nurse to provide collaborative care based on the highest standards, knowledge and competence.
2: Knowing Ourselves Acknowledge your strengths and challenges and recognize how you can build on these for your future Explore the way you respond to challenges and acknowledge this as a way of managing strange situations	Professional Values	**1.7** All nurses must be responsible and accountable for keeping their knowledge and skills up to date through continuing professional development. They must aim to improve their performance and enhance the safety of care through evaluation, supervision and appraisal.	**Care, Compassion and Communication**	**3.** People can trust the newly registered graduate nurse to respect them as individuals and strive to help them preserve their dignity at all times.

(Continued)

Chapter number, title and learning outcomes	NMC Standards for Pre-registration Nursing Education (2010)		Essential skills cluster	
	Domain	Competency	Cluster	Skill
Identify your beliefs and values as a professional practitioner Understand your learning style and how this influences the way in which you learn Identify your attitudes to writing and your writing style.		**1.8** All nurses must practice independently, recognizing the limits of their competence and knowledge. They must **reflect** on these limits and seek advice from, or refer to, other professionals where necessary.	**Care, Compassion and Communication**	**5.** People can trust the newly registered nurse to engage with them in a warm, sensitive and compassionate way.
	Communication and interpersonal skills	**5.1** Mental health nurses must use their personal qualities, experiences and interpersonal skills to develop and maintain therapeutic, recovery-focused relationships with people and therapeutic groups. They must be aware of their own mental health, and know when to share aspects of their own life to inspire hope while maintaining professional boundaries.		**6.** People can trust the newly registered nurse to engage therapeutically and actively listen to their needs and concerns, responding using skills that are helpful, providing information that is clear, meaningful and free from jargon.
	Leadership, management and team working	**4.4** All nurses must be **self-aware** and recognize how their values, principles and assumptions may affect their practice. They must maintain their own personal and professional development, learning from experience, through supervision, feedback, **reflection** and evaluation.	**Organizational Aspects of Care**	**18.** People can trust a newly registered graduate nurse to enhance the safety of service users and identify and actively manage risk and uncertainty in relation to people, the environment, self and others.

Chapter	Domain	Standard	Essential Skills Cluster	
3: Frameworks for Reflection Recognize and utilize some frameworks for reflection Work through some of your own experiences using these frameworks Create 'model' critical incident analyses from your own experience.	**Professional Values**	**1.7** All nurses must be responsible and accountable for keeping their knowledge and skills up to date through continuing professional development. They must aim to improve their performance and enhance the safety of care through evaluation, supervision and appraisal.	**Care, Compassion and Communication**	**7.** People can trust the newly registered nurse to protect and keep as confidential all information relating to them.
	Leadership, management and team working	**1.8** All nurses must practice independently, recognizing the limits of their competence and knowledge. They must **reflect** on these limits and seek advice from, or refer to, other professionals where necessary. **4.4** All nurses must be **self-aware** and recognize how their values, principles and assumptions may affect their practice. They must maintain their own personal and professional development, learning from experience, through supervision, feedback, **reflection** and evaluation.	**Organizational Aspects of Care**	**10.** People can trust the newly registered graduate nurse to deliver nursing interventions and evaluate their effectiveness against the agreed assessment and care plan.
4: Entering the Working Environment Consider your role as a student in the working environment Anticipate the challenges of entering different working environments	**Professional Values**	**1.1** All nurses must practice with confidence according to The Code: Standards of Conduct, performance and Ethics for nurses and midwives (NMC 2008) and within other recognized ethical and legal frameworks.	**Organizational Aspects of Care**	**11.** People can trust the newly registered graduate nurse to safeguard children and adults from vulnerable situations and support and protect them from harm.

(Continued)

Chapter number, title and learning outcomes	NMC Standards for Pre-registration Nursing Education (2010)		Essential skills cluster	
	Domain	Competency	Cluster	Skill
Understand the need to plan your learning experiences in practice to achieve competencies Consider the role of other people in your learning in practice.		**1.7** All nurses must be responsible and accountable for keeping their knowledge and skills up to date through continuing professional development. They must aim to improve their performance and enhance the safety of care through evaluation, supervision and appraisal. **1.8** All nurses must practice independently, recognizing the limits of their competence and knowledge. They must **reflect** on these limits and seek advice from, or refer to, other professionals where necessary.		**12.** People can trust the newly registered graduate nurse to respond to their feedback and a wide range of other sources to learn, develop and improve services.
	Nursing practice and decision-making	**1.** All nurses must use up to date knowledge and evidence to assess, plan, deliver and evaluate care, communicate findings, influence change and promote health and best practice. They must make person-centred, evidence-based judgments and decisions, in partnership with others involved in the care process, to ensure high quality care. They must be able to recognize when the complexity of clinical decisions requires specialist knowledge and expertise and consult or refer accordingly.		

Chapter		Standards for competence	Essential skills clusters	
		10. All nurses must evaluate their care to improve clinical decision-making, quality and outcomes, using a range of methods, amending the plan of care where necessary and communicating changes to others.	**Care, Compassion and Communication**	**1.** As partners in the care process, people can trust a newly registered graduate nurse to provide collaborative care based on the highest standards, knowledge and competence.
	Leadership, management and team working	**4.4** All nurses must be **self-aware** and recognize how their values, principles and assumptions may affect their practice. They must maintain their own personal and professional development, learning from experience, through supervision, feedback, **reflection** and evaluation.		
5: Ways of reflecting on your own Identify ways of reflecting that suit your learning style Explore a range of reflective strategies that can be used for personal reflection Identify the differences between written reflective strategies and other ways of reflecting Consider the ways in which you can use reflective writing within your portfolio.	**Professional Values**	**1.7** All nurses must be responsible and accountable for keeping their knowledge and skills up to date through continuing professional development. They must aim to improve their performance and enhance the safety of care through evaluation, supervision and appraisal. **1.8** All nurses must practice independently, recognizing the limits of their competence and knowledge. They must **reflect** on these limits and seek advice from, or refer to, other professionals where necessary.	**Organizational Aspects of Care**	**12.** People can trust the newly registered graduate nurse to respond to their feedback and a wide range of other sources to learn, develop and improve services.

(Continued)

Chapter number, title and learning outcomes	NMC Standards for Pre-registration Nursing Education (2010)			Essential skills cluster	
	Domain	Competency		Cluster	Skill
6: Ways of reflecting with others Identify the benefits of reflecting with others Explore issues that need careful thinking about before reflecting with others Identify ways of reflecting with your peers, colleagues and friends Discuss the use of reflection with clinical mentors, assessors and other professional groups Explore the use of reflective strategies with educational staff.	**Professional Values**	**1.1** All nurses must practice with confidence according to The Code: Standards of Conduct, performance and Ethics for nurses and midwives (NMC 2008) and within other recognized ethical and legal frameworks. **1.7** All nurses must be responsible and accountable for keeping their knowledge and skills up to date through continuing professional development. They must aim to improve their performance and enhance the safety of care through evaluation, supervision and appraisal. **1.8** All nurses must practice independently, recognizing the limits of their competence and knowledge. They must **reflect** on these limits and seek advice from, or refer to, other professionals where necessary.		**Care, Compassion and Communication** **Organizational Aspects of Care**	**1.** As partners in the care process, people can trust a newly registered graduate nurse to provide collaborative care based on the highest standards, knowledge and competence. **7.** People can trust the newly registered nurse to protect and keep as confidential all information relating to them. **11.** People can trust the newly registered graduate nurse to safeguard children and adults from vulnerable situations and support and protect them from harm.

Communication and interpersonal skills	**5.1** Mental health nurses must use their personal qualities, experiences and interpersonal skills to develop and maintain therapeutic, recovery-focused relationships with people and therapeutic groups. They must be aware of their own mental health, and know when to share aspects of their own life to inspire hope while maintaining professional boundaries.	**12.** People can trust the newly registered graduate nurse to respond to their feedback and a wide range of other sources to learn, develop and improve services.
Leadership, management and team working	**4.4** All nurses must be **self-aware** and recognize how their values, principles and assumptions may affect their practice. They must maintain their own personal and professional development, learning from experience, through supervision, feedback, **reflection** and evaluation.	**18.** People can trust a newly registered graduate nurse to enhance the safety of service users and identify and actively manage risk and uncertainty in relation to people, the environment, self and others.

RAPID RECAP ANSWERS

CHAPTER 1

1 **What is the ERA cycle of reflective practice?**

    Experience–reflection–action

2 **What are Schön's two types of reflection?**

    Reflection-in-action and reflection-on-action

3 **What is the difference between the reflective processes and reflective practice?**

    Reflective practice requires some sort of action to be taken

4 **What are the stages in the reflective processes?**

    The stages of the reflective processes are:

    Stage 1: Selecting a critical incident to reflect on
    Stage 2: Observing and describing the experience
    Stage 3: Analyzing the experience
    Stage 4: Interpreting the experience
    Stage 5: Exploring alternatives.
    Stage 6: Framing action

5 **What is meant by the term 'critical incident'?**

    A critical incident is an event that stands out in your mind and contributes directly to developing as a practitioner

CHAPTER 2

1 **What is a SWOB analysis?**

    A SWOB analysis is a way of identifying your strengths and weaknesses, the opportunities that you have and the barriers to achieving these

2 **Where do our professional values come from?**

Professional values come from a variety of sources including:

- Received from external sources – media, people we know, careers information
- Our own personality, attitudes and approach to life, and cultural experiences
- Other professionals
- Generally accepted beliefs and moral codes
- Codes of professional conduct

3 **How can knowing your preferred learning style help you to learn more effectively?**

Recognizing the ways in which we learn helps us to select methods that we will benefit from most

4 **What are the challenges to using writing to learn?**

Challenges might be:

- Overcoming the rules for writing
- Writing for ourselves instead of others
- Using the features of the 'writing-to-learn' paradigm
- Overcoming the need to 'get it right'
- Completing the reflective cycle
- Deciding on the difference between public and private writing
- Anticipating the consequences of our writing
- Finding something to write about
- Getting started

CHAPTER 3

1 **What are Goodman's three levels of reflection?**

First level – reflection to reach given objectives
Second level – reflection on the relationship between principles and practice
Third level – reflection that, besides the above, incorporates ethical and political concerns

2 **What are the six stages of Gibbs's reflective cycle?**

Description, feelings, evaluation, analysis, conclusions, action planning

3 **What might be a drawback to using Gibbs's cycle within reflective practice?**

It stops at the end of the reflective processes and does not proceed to the 'taking action' stage of the ERA cycle.

4 **What are the main differences between Gibbs's and Johns' frameworks?**

Gibbs	Johns
The framework arose from education	The model arose from clinical practice
It focuses on the experience itself	It focuses on uncovering the knowledge behind the experience
It is a reflective cycle consisting of six stages	It has a core question and a series of cue questions
It focuses on learning from the incident	It focuses on the practitioner's intentions and actions
It focuses on the individual's actions	It incorporates the actions of others present

5 **What are Carper's types of knowing?**

Empirics, ethics, personal, aesthetics

6 **What are Borton's three cue questions?**

What? So what? Now what?

CHAPTER 4

1 **What is the primary difference between the college environment and the practice environment?**

The college's purpose is education; whereas the primary purpose in practice is to deliver a health care service to the public.

2 **To whom do you have responsibilities in the clinical environment?**

To yourself; to patients and their carers; to other staff and colleagues.

3 **What are your roles as a student in the practice environment?**

To learn to be a safe and competent professional practitioner; to deliver care; to work as a team member.

4 **What is meant by 'self-empowerment'?**

Taking responsibility for your own actions and enabling yourself to achieve for the future.

5 **What are the different types of learning opportunities available in clinical practice?**

Learning from others; learning from different clinical placements; learning from events; learning through achievement of course competencies and learning outcomes; learning from your own interests and needs.

6 **What is meant by the term 'socialization processes'?**

How we learn to fit into different social situations and function within our profession. They include the language we use, the ways in which we work, our attitudes, skills and professional attributes.

7 **How can we get the most out of the opportunities available for learning in practice?**

By taking the time to reflect, analyze and plan.

CHAPTER 5

1 **What is the difference between reflection-in-action and reflection-on-action?**

Reflection-in-action occurs while we are doing things and is largely unconscious. Reflection-on-action occurs after the event and is a deliberate activity.

2 **What is reflective writing?**

Reflective writing is writing for the purpose of learning from your experiences and identifying future action.

3 **What are the features of reflective writing?**

We write reflectively to:

- Achieve a purpose
- Order our thoughts
- Create a permanent record
- Be creative
- Develop our analytical skills
- Develop our critical thinking
- Develop new understandings and knowledge
- Show that we understand something.

4 **What are the two categories of reflective writing?**

Analytical and creative.

5 **How can you plan to write safely?**

Safe writing involves:

- Setting your own rules
- Establishing the purpose of your reflection
- Selecting your own models and frameworks
- Retaining control over who sees your writing and what they see
- Storing it in a safe place
- Planning to complete the reflective cycle.

CHAPTER 6

1 **What are the benefits of reflecting with others?**

They can take a more objective stance to something that has happened to you:

- They may ask questions that you have not thought of yourself
- They may offer a different way of seeing things
- They can act as a sounding board for your ideas
- They can validate your thoughts about a situation
- They may help you to put events into a different context
- They bring their own knowledge and experiences to the situation which may help your understanding
- They may offer alternative courses of action to those you have come up with.

2 **What different groups of people could you choose to reflect with?**

Family, friends and colleagues; staff in the clinical environment; educational staff.

3 **What issues do you need to think about before starting to reflect with others?**

To establish the purpose of the encounter; to consider the nature of the relationship; to set boundaries and ground rules; to consider the risks of reflecting with others; to consider the professional and ethical implications.

4 **How can you make the most of reflecting with others?**

- We can use the different relationships that we have with others for different kinds of reflection, remembering that one-to-one reflection has a different nature from group reflection.
- Forward planning before any reflective encounter with others will ensure that our own needs are met.
- Remember that the primary responsibility for the student's learning within reflective encounters lies with the student.

INDEX